The Feisty Woman's Breast Cancer Book

FOR REBECCA

Ordering

Trade bookstores in the U.S. and Canada please contact:

Publishers Group West
1700 Fourth Street, Berkeley, CA 94710
Phone: (800) 788-3123   Fax: (510) 528-3444

Hunter House books are available at bulk discounts for textbook course adoptions; to qualifying community, healthcare, and government organizations; and for special promotions and fundraising. For details please contact:

Special Sales Department
Hunter House Inc., PO Box 2914, Alameda CA 94501-0914
Tel. (510) 865-5282   Fax (510) 865-4295
e-mail: ordering@hunterhouse.com

Individuals can order our books from most bookstores or by calling toll-free:
1-800-266-5592

For related information on this book, visit the author's website at:
www.feistywoman.com

The Feisty Woman's Breast Cancer Book

by Elaine Ratner

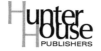
Hunter House
PUBLISHERS

Copyright © 1999 by Elaine Ratner

Hunter House Inc., Publishers
P.O. Box 2914
Alameda CA 94501-0914

Library of Congress Cataloging-in-Publication Data
Ratner, Elaine.
The feisty woman's breast cancer book / by Elaine Ratner. – 1st ed.
    p.   cm.
Includes bibliographical references.
ISBN 0-89793-270-6 (cloth). – ISBN 0-89793-269-2 (paper)
1.   Breast – Cancer – Psychological aspects. 2. Breast – Cancer
Popular works. I. Title
RC280.B8R38 1999   99-23722
616.99'449—dc21   CIP

Project credits

Cover Design: Knockout Design   *Book Design/Production:* Brian Dittmar
Developmental Editor: Laura Harger   *Copy Editor:* Kristi Hein
Managing Editor: Wendy Low   *Editorial Assistant:* Jennifer Rader
Acquisitions: Jeanne Brondino   *Editorial Intern:* Rachel McMillan
Proofreader: Lee Rappold   *Indexer:* Kathy Talley-Jones
Publicity Director: Marisa Spatafore   *Publisher's Assistant:* Georgia Moseley
Customer Service Manager: Christina Sverdrup
Order Fulfillment: Joel Irons, A & A Quality Shipping Services
Publisher: Kiran S. Rana

Printed and bound by Publisher's Press, Salt Lake City, UT
Manufactured in the United States of America

9 8 7 6 5 4 3 2 1   First Edition   99 00 01 02 03

Contents

Acknowledgments

A great many people helped to make this book possible. Before I even knew there would be a book, there was breast cancer, and all the people who helped me to cope. First and foremost, my husband and daughter, Jay and Rebecca Harlow. They were there for me every step of the way; their love fueled my determination to recover.

My friends were there too, giving generously of their time and supporting me in countless ways. Thanks to Gerry Dunn and Steve Gerardin, Tim Ware and Kim Davenport, Susan Mattmann and Matt Morse, Darol Anger and Willa Rabinovitch, Mike Marshall and Kaila Flexer, Alison Odell and Julian Smedley, Sally Shepard, Dayna Macy, Dan McClain, Francine Halberg, and Barbara Tropp. And my heartfelt thanks to the doctors in the surgery department at Kaiser Hospital, without whose persistence and skill I might not be here today.

As I struggled to turn my breast cancer experience into a breast cancer book, my husband Jay was a constant source of help and encouragement. He took over more of our business to give me time to write and read and discussed every draft of every chapter, and still insisted he loved being married to me.

As the book took shape, other friends read parts or all of it and gave me invaluable feedback. Thanks to Marilyn Aiches, Kim Davenport, Gerry Dunn, Phoebe Harlow, Rhonda Hughes, Nancy Lucas, Dayna Macy, Sally and Jim Shepard, and Luke Szpakowski. Margo Perin, who read the manuscript while preparing for her own breast cancer surgery, gave the book its first road test; her enthusiastic response erased some of my lingering doubts.

Thanks also to Terry Odean, for his patient explanations of the way statistics work, and to Sheryl Fullerton, whose early interest in the project helped me believe it would one day be published. Positive feedback from others in the book trade, including Elizabeth Whipple, Michael Korda, Julie Bennett, Rux Martin, and Karen Cross, kept me moving forward.

Finally, special thanks to the folks at Hunter House, who have been an absolute pleasure to work with, especially Jeanne Brondino, who read the manuscript first and took it under her wing, and Kiran Rana, who welcomed it. Thanks also to Jennifer Rader, Wendy Low, Marisa Spatafore, and my editor, Laura Harger. You've helped me to fulfill a dream.

Introduction

Before I discovered two malignant lumps in my breast in the spring of 1995, I had very little experience with being ill. I began my encounter with breast cancer with all the trepidation you would expect in a woman suddenly facing a dreaded and potentially fatal disease. To my amazement, my medical experience was nowhere near as awful as I feared it would be. I had found my cancer while it was still in an early, treatable stage. I have since discovered that most women do.

While we all imagine that every woman with breast cancer is facing death or dreadful disfigurement, most are actually more in danger of being scarred by the psychological and emotional impact of the disease, its treatments, and the attitudes of our culture toward women's breasts. Yet when it comes to offering guidance in those critical areas, most doctors and books on cancer are either silent or hopelessly off base. As a woman with breast cancer, I had to pinpoint and resolve the psychological and emotional problems for myself. Looking back, I realize how much a little bit of wise counsel would have meant to me.

Here is a list of the things I wish someone had told me at the beginning of my breast cancer experience:

- ✓ A breast is completely expendable.
- ✓ You may die of breast cancer, but you probably won't.
- ✓ There is enough time.
- ✓ Worry makes things worse.
- ✓ Surround yourself with people who make you feel good.
- ✓ Don't shut out your family, especially children.
- ✓ Think about all you have to live for.
- ✓ It's important to know what's important to you.
- ✓ Insist on a doctor you trust.
- ✓ Nobody really knows much about breast cancer.

✓ Try anything that might help.

✓ Expectations influence outcome.

✓ The human body is a miraculous healing machine.

✓ A one-breasted body isn't ugly, just different.

✓ Losing a breast doesn't have to affect your sex life.

✓ Wisdom and strength are aftereffects of breast cancer.

✓ If you want things to change, you have to speak up.

✓ We all need to change our attitudes toward women's breasts.

These eighteen points—insights, you might call them—became the inspiration for the chapters of this book.

This is the book I searched for when I was facing breast cancer, but never found. It is not a book of medical facts, or a political call to arms, or a diary of a brave woman's struggle against a terrifying disease. There are lots of those on the market already. I read many of them, and found some helpful. But they did not answer the questions that were most important to me. They did not tell me how to hold on emotionally and psychologically during my medical ordeal so that, whatever happened to my body, as a person I would emerge healthy and whole. During my breast cancer experience and in the four years since, I have explored my basic beliefs about love and friendship, self-confidence and self-consciousness, health and beauty, both real and perceived. The questions I asked myself and the answers I ultimately arrived at are laid out here.

I am well aware that my questions may not be your questions, and my answers may not be your answers. That is as it should be. When it comes to matters of health and love, we must all decide for ourselves. I do not expect—or want—you to take my answers, or my decisions, and make them your own. I hope, instead, that my experience will encourage you to pursue your own answers and make your own decisions with confidence.

One thing I learned for certain through having breast cancer is that feistiness is good for your health. As our system of medical care has become increasingly "managed," it has gotten harder for doctors to give each patient all the time they would like to give, and harder for patients to get the attention, and sometimes the treatments, they feel they need. Feisty patients—those who speak up loud and clear, who politely but firmly demand the information they need to make important medical decisions, and who insist that the medical system respect their right to make those decisions—are far more likely to get first-rate care than those who are timid.

What's more, there is mounting medical evidence that patients who are feisty and take action on their own behalf are more likely to survive a serious illness, and more likely to fully recover, than patients who are passive and accepting. This is equally true of male and female patients, but it's often harder for women to be bold and outspoken. It takes practice, so I encourage you to start practicing now.

Whether your breast cancer experience is limited to monthly self-exams and a yearly mammogram or balloons into a full-blown medical ordeal, I hope this book will make it easier to handle. I have tried to expose misinformation that scared me, so that you will be less scared. I have tried to explain insights that took months for me to arrive at, so that you can have them sooner, to accept or reject as you see fit. And I have tried to emphasize the positive aspects of my experience, because writers in the health field too often forget to mention the good things that can come from experiencing a life-threatening illness.

If you are now facing breast cancer, you may not believe that good things can come from it. I didn't either. And yet here I am, four years later, a healthier, happier, better-adjusted woman than I was before breast cancer entered my life. I hope that four years from today, you will be saying the same thing.

Elaine Ratner
FEBRUARY 1999

Free Yourself from the Breast Myth

A breast is completely expendable.

As a society we are obsessed with women's breasts. As women, we are being hurt by that obsession, in more ways and in more devastating ways than we realize. Worship of the female breast influences not only our fashion choices, but our medical choices as well, especially those having to do with breast cancer. We cannot hope to deal rationally with the threat of breast cancer, as individuals or as a community, until we demystify the female breast and learn to see it for what it is: a body part that has an important function and is certainly pleasing, but is neither the source of our femininity nor the seat of our emotional well-being, and is certainly not the reason we are loved....

Until I was struck with breast cancer, I didn't spend a lot of time thinking about breasts. Mine were one of the few parts of my body that I considered acceptable, so I tucked them into a bra every morning and let them be. For years, while millions of other women were buying push-up bras or having silicone bags inserted in their breasts to make them bigger and more upstanding, I was fixating on my heavy thighs and increasingly flabby upper arms. Locked in my personal self-torture chamber, I was more or less oblivious to the latest rise of the female breast in popular culture.

To be honest, I was just as oblivious to most other trends in popular culture. I don't watch much television, have never had cable, and seldom have time to read magazines that don't relate to my work. When I read the morning newspaper, I ignore the ads unless I'm in the market for a particular item, and then I read only the ads that pertain to that product. Not being in the market for new and improved breasts, and occupied with trying to fill all my responsibilities as a wife, mother, and business owner, I went through my harried days hardly noticing that all around me female breasts were getting bigger and more prominent.

Then cancer took a hand, and my attention zoomed in on female breasts. Suddenly I noticed that breasts were everywhere. They poked out at me from the covers of magazines in supermarket racks. They basked in the spotlight in commercials, movies, and the television sitcoms my daughter watches before dinner. They rumbled by on the mud flaps of big rig trucks and called out from calendars piled on bookstore tables before Christmas. It was as if I had woken from a long sleep. I felt like a contemporary Rip van Winkle, blinking and staring and wondering how I'd missed so major a phenomenon for so long.

The reason for my sudden sensitivity to breasts, of course, was that my own breasts had become the focus of my life. The nicely shaped, size 36-C breasts that I had benignly ignored for years grabbed center stage on a Sunday night in April 1995, just a couple of weeks past my fifty-first birthday. I was standing at the sink brushing my teeth. As I reached for a towel, my hand accidentally brushed against my left breast and felt a lump. In that instant I felt the grip of fear. You do feel it—cold and kind of stiff, squeezing your whole body, not hard, but firmly, unmistakably.

As I stood, momentarily immobilized, I could feel the focus of my life shift. All of my energy, my thoughts, and, most of all, my fears turned toward my breast. All at once it was my center. It was me.

It would be two months before that lump, and a second one that turned up beside it, were definitively diagnosed as cancer. But on that cool April night, standing alone in my bathroom, I knew I was in trouble. That night I joined the millions of American women and men who are obsessed with breasts.

A Dangerous Obsession

One of the reasons breast cancer is so terrifyingly powerful—far out of proportion to the health threat the disease actually represents—is that the part of the body it attacks is a highly charged symbol. The female breast has always been prominent in the mythologies that have shaped civilization. In the ancient goddess cultures, it symbolized the earth mother, the source of life, power, and wisdom. Such female deities were long ago dethroned, but in the male-dominated religions and cultures that followed, the female breast remained a powerful symbol, prominent in paintings, sculpture, and the minds of the public. Through the ages the image of the female breast has been called upon to stir emotional support for a wide range of cultural values, including religious martyrdom, national allegiance, and maternal devotion. [1] These days it is used mainly to stir male sexual desire. The popular culture that has become our modern mythology—shaping our lives more than most of us would care to admit—does its best to ignore both the breast's powerful history and its nurturing function. Our icons are not earth mothers any more, but nubile actresses and models. The female breast is now a symbol not of our connection to the earth or to each other, but of our endless pursuit of beauty, youth, and sexuality.

Our contemporary culture still worships the female body. We have simply narrowed our admiration for it to a single feature, its ability to attract and please men. We measure its power by cup size. Our modern mythology tells men that a woman with large and shapely breasts is the ultimate prize, and that possessing her is proof of superior manhood. It tells women that voluptuous breasts will assure us popularity, and much more. They are the essence of our femininity, it insists, the very foundation of the female ego.

If we stop to think for a moment, it becomes obvious that the current emphasis on large breasts is just a fashion. In other times, and not so long ago, flat-chested women were the beauty ideal. Remember the flappers? Remember Jackie Kennedy? Remember Twiggy?

It seems every decade has its particular marks of beauty upon which the popular culture bestows its seal of approval by declaring them sexy. When I was in college, long, straight hair was so honored, and I remember the fashion-conscious coeds in my dorm bent over ironing boards in our basement laundry room, ironing out each other's curl. It was silly, perhaps, but essentially harmless. Today, the two female features considered most "sexy" seriously threaten our health. The quest for extreme thinness keeps millions of women on dangerous diets and diet pills, and sends countless teenage girls down the road to anorexia and bulimia. The worship of big breasts sends healthy women into surgery. In the last 20 years, more than a million American women have had their breasts surgically enlarged, convinced that bigger breasts would make them more attractive to men and make them feel better about themselves. Unfortunately, many who sought to improve their social lives and self-image by implanting bags of silicone in their breasts developed serious health problems they believe stemmed from leaking implants. Hundreds of thousands have sued the implant manufacturers. [2]

Despite all the well-publicized health problems, at some level we all wish we looked more like the shapely female celebrities set out for us to envy in movies, on television, and in magazines. Oh, we know they are the creations of makeup artists, carefully controlled lighting, and perfect camera angles. We know that most of them achieve their ultra-slim, overly buxom bodies through starvation, hours-long daily workouts with expensive trainers, and, often, plastic surgery. Still, it's hard to keep from being drawn into the fantasy settings in which these "ideal" women perform; it's hard not to wonder whether, if we looked like them, we too could attract the attention of gorgeous men and add a bit more excitement and glamour to our lives.

Whether achieving the sought-after shape is even possible for most women soon becomes beside the point. Once a woman accepts the look as a cultural ideal, it affects her life, and distorts her self-image. It even influences those of us who try to ignore popular culture. It is as if all the mirrors in America come from the factory with the current image of ideal female beauty outlined on their surface. When we stand before them, we can't help seeing that we don't quite fit its contours. Everyone looks too short or too tall or too fat or too thin; nobody's face is pretty enough, and nobody's breasts look right.

When breast cancer entered my life, the way I looked at my body suddenly changed. I stopped worrying about its size and shape, and began worrying about whether it would survive. When I stood in front of my mirror, instead of focusing on the outer flaws it reflected, I searched for signs of strength and courage beneath the surface. As I moved through breast cancer diagnosis and treatment, I gradually rejected popular assumptions about "how women feel" and "what women want" and replaced them with what this woman actually felt and wanted. Each time I swept aside an expectation that didn't fit me, the image in my mirror seemed clearer, and more pleasing.

But I am getting ahead of my story. When I first discovered a lump in my breast, I didn't think about popular culture, or superficial images of women, or the pressure to conform. My mind was focused on just two things: I was afraid of dying, and I was afraid of losing my breast.

Confronting Breast Cancer and Myself
◎

Early on the morning after I found my lump I was at my HMO. The nurse practitioner who examined my breast felt not just one lump, but two, and sent me immediately for a mammogram. Knowing next to nothing about breast cancer diagnosis, I naively thought the mammogram would tell the story. I gathered my courage and steeled myself for the news.

It turns out that mammograms are far from definitive. Mine showed that something was happening in my breast, all right, but although several specialists consulted on the reading, no one was certain just what it was. A few days later, a young surgical resident tried to explain to me all the different conditions that could cause the ominous dark areas on my x-ray, some of them dangerous, some not. The idea began to sink in that I was going to have to live with uncertainty, and my fears, much longer than I had expected.

The next test was a sonogram, which uses sound waves to determine if a lump is solid or filled with fluid. Fluid is good; it means a lump is not cancer. Solid may be bad, or it may not be.

On the day of my sonogram I was nervous. Weeks had passed, and I was anxious to have an answer. The technician who conducted the test was pleasant and polite until she started moving her sensor around on my bare breast. Then she became annoyingly silent. She sat watching a little screen, saying absolutely nothing. I tried to pry something out of her.

"What do you see?" I asked.

"I'm not supposed to say," was her answer. Hospital policy kept her lips sealed. I had to wait, again, for a doctor to give me the news.

Waiting for my next appointment, I tried to keep my normal life going. I sat through business meetings, had my hair cut, reported for jury duty. But a part of me was always focused on my breast, wondering, worrying, wishing I knew what was coming.

As it turned out, the sonogram, too, was inconclusive. It showed that the lumps were not filled with fluid. That meant they could be cancer or could be something harmless. The young resident seemed confident that I didn't have cancer. The lumps felt rounded, he said, not jagged on the edges, and they moved easily under his fingers. Those were good signs. He tried to reassure me, and I tried to believe him, but the slowness and uncertainty of the diagnostic process were taking their toll.

The sonogram was followed by a needle aspiration, the actual removal of cells for examination. It took a week to get results, which were also inconclusive. I was told the next step would be a surgical biopsy, in which my lumps would be removed and sent to a pathology lab for analysis. Two months had passed, and the main thing I had learned was how to live with not knowing. In retrospect, it was an important lesson.

Dr. R., an oncological surgeon, performed the biopsy. A week later he told me that both of my lumps were malignant and I needed a mastectomy. When I asked what my alternatives were, he said I had no choice. I accepted his medical judgment, but I rebelled against the "no choice" part. I was also annoyed that during our short consultation he kept using medical terminology I didn't understand. I had to stop him repeatedly to ask for explanations. I felt he was treating me like a child, or like someone too scared and upset to make responsible decisions. He, and other medical staff, no longer saw me as a woman undergoing tests. They now saw me as an official "breast cancer patient." Suddenly I sensed that everyone at the hospital believed I was headed for a major psychological crisis, and therefore required special handling.

My HMO is so worried about the mental state of breast cancer patients that the surgery department has a full-time "breast care coordinator," a nurse whose entire job is to help women with breast cancer to adjust. A few minutes after Dr. R. broke the news, I was ushered into her office for moral support. She was sympathetic and kind, but her concern reinforced my feeling that my emotional reactions were being closely watched. She suggested I get a second surgeon's opinion, and I agreed, not because I doubted Dr. R.'s diagnosis, but because I was suddenly uncomfortable with him. An oncologist friend recommended another surgeon in the same department, and the following week my husband and I went together to meet Dr. S.

As is typical in medical situations, the conversation was not set up to be a discussion between equals. I was sitting on an examining table, my chest bare under a blue plastic vest that had no ties to keep it closed. Under me, protecting the table, was a strip of white paper. My feet dangled several inches above the floor. Tall and burly and fully clothed, Dr. S. stood looking at me with a serious, steady gaze.

I found his manner a bit paternalistic, but I liked his forceful personality and his high energy level. I also liked the fact that he spoke to me in plain English. He made it clear that he thought a mastectomy was my best bet. "If you were my wife ..." he intoned, in a manner I have since learned is not unusual for male surgeons to use. *I'm not your wife*, I thought, but I knew he was probably right. Still, he offered me an alternative: instead of a mastectomy, I could have a lumpectomy followed by radiation. He added that he would press Dr. R. to provide the lesser operation if that's what I wanted.

That wasn't what I wanted. I just wanted a doctor who would talk honestly with me, then let me make my own decisions. I decided then and there to have the mastectomy and I asked Dr. S. to perform it.

Psyche in Peril
❁

With our primary business taken care of, he turned his attention to what he, too, obviously considered my imperiled psyche. He wanted me to follow the mastectomy with breast reconstruction surgery. To his credit, he prefaced his pitch for reconstruction by saying, "There is no medical reason to do this." Still, he tried hard to persuade me. "We have found that women do not heal well psychologically after mastectomy unless they have reconstruction," he told me. He didn't ask me how I felt about the prospect of losing a breast.

Sitting there in that ridiculous plastic vest, I felt vulnerable and small. Visions of Nazi medical experiments I had heard about as a child in Sunday School flashed across my mind, and I knew I could never let anyone plant a foreign object inside my chest. I said flatly that I didn't want reconstruction, and Dr. S. backed off, temporarily.

Afterward, I kept wondering why he had brought up reconstruction at all. Here I was—facing major surgery, the loss of my breast, and perhaps the ravages of a fatal disease—and my surgeon, instead of concentrating on saving my life, was talking about my appearance. Couldn't he at least wait until he knew if I was going to survive?

My cynical side wondered whether he had financial motives in pushing me toward cosmetic surgery. But that thought didn't last long. As an oncological surgeon, he doesn't do plastic surgery himself, and I doubt that the nonprofit HMO he works for gives bonuses for referring patients to its plastic surgeon. No, I am certain that he recommended reconstructive surgery because he truly believed I would not recover as well without it. *He doesn't know me at all*, I kept thinking. *How can he know how I'm going to feel when I don't even know?*

The Breast Myth Affects Us All

Like everyone else in our society, surgeons are affected by popular culture. They, like most of the rest of us, have been convinced that a woman's self-image is centered in her breasts. Perhaps, because they believe that to be true, they worry that they are destroying their breast cancer patients psychologically by the very act they perform to save them physically. If so, they are carrying a heavy psychological burden themselves and are as much victims of the breast myth as the women who are their patients.

As I look back on my breast cancer experience, I have many times wished that instead of being negative and predicting certain psychological pain, Dr. S. had been positive and reassured me that such pain is unnecessary. I wish that, instead of pushing reconstruction as my only hope for psychological healing, he had said that a woman could get along fine with just one breast. I wish he had told me that day some of the things it took months for me to figure out for myself—such as the fact that a woman's breasts are external, and that from a health point of view they are completely expendable.

I consider myself fortunate that my cancer was in my breast. If it had been in a lung, that would have been far worse. If it had been in an ovary or my cervix, I would have had to undergo much more serious and dangerous surgery. If it had been in my bones, or my brain, or my pancreas, or my throat … I think any of those would have been a nightmare. But my cancer was in my breast—my external, expendable breast—and that was a blessing.

When I talk now to a woman worried about losing a breast, I always point out that she doesn't need a breast to live well. A breast doesn't pump your blood or digest your food. You don't breathe with it or use it to walk or talk. As I say those things I can usually feel attitudes changing. "I'm so glad you said that," several women have said to me. "I never thought about it that way."

Despite all the hype about women's breasts, the truth is that unless she's determined to breast-feed, a woman simply doesn't need them. Don't get me wrong, they're nice to have, but you don't need them. If I had to choose a part of my body to sacrifice, a breast would be my first choice. Before a finger or a big toe. No other body part is as expendable. Recognizing that fact was the most positive and most important insight of my breast cancer experience—and one that took months to become clear.

My Breast Is Not Me

In the weeks between my diagnosis and my mastectomy, my mind wandered frequently to thoughts of surgery and how losing a breast would forever change me. I would stop what I was doing and sit still, waiting to be engulfed by emotion. I'd look down at my left breast, trying to feel the sense of loss I was sure would come. It never came. Not that I was too numb to feel; whenever I thought about the possibility of dying, a chilling fear swooped down on me. I felt it in every cell of my body. I just couldn't stir up any bad feelings about losing my breast. After a while, I stopped expecting them.

Although I was not worried about losing a breast, I expected to be unnerved by the sight of my chest after mastectomy. I was sure I would feel depressed by my scars and lopsidedness and that I would hate the new shape of my body. Knowing that I could not face reconstruction, I told myself I would have to learn to live with my appearance, no matter how bad it was.

A week after the mastectomy, I returned to the hospital to have my bandages removed. Dr. S. yanked out the tubes that had been draining my chest. I looked down and saw metal staples, about thirty in all, in a neat line. I had assumed there would be stitches. I was shocked. I looked like something out of a horror film, a female Frankenstein's monster. I was also surprised to see that except for the staples, the left side of my chest looked smooth and calm.

Many times in the following week I pulled off my shirt and stood in front of the mirror. Instead of being repelled by what I saw, I was fascinated. Who would have thought you could put a human body together with staples? I decided the onslaught of negative emotions would come once the staples were removed and I would be able to see my body as it was going to be.

Another week passed, and the staples came out. The incision scar was already healed. It was pink and as thin as a pencil line, and it flowed gracefully across my chest. On either side was a row of tiny perpendicular lines marking the places where the staples had been.

I continued my daily ritual of standing in front of the mirror, trying to feel whatever it was I was going to feel. The wrong feelings kept coming up. I would look at my lopsided chest and feel pleasure. No, I would think, that's not right. So I would do my best to sweep the feeling away and wait for it to be replaced by something more properly negative. But as I looked at my chest, with its nicely shaped breast on one side and a smooth, slightly undulating surface on the other, I kept thinking in spite of myself, "That's kind of cool."

I examined the left side of my torso carefully and decided it looked like the torso of a young man. I argued with myself about his age. Late teens—no, early twenties. I thought about male models in bathing suits and compared my look to theirs. About 21, I decided. My left side was that of a 21-year-old male, not yet maturely muscled, but certainly no longer a boy. And on the right side I was a mature, rather nicely endowed woman. I was androgynous, unconventional, interesting, and attractive. I liked my new body, and I was amazed that I liked it.

I began to think that symmetry is overrated. Looking like everyone else is fine, but looking different is more intriguing. I remember thinking that Renoir, for years my favorite painter, is wonderful, but Picasso has more vitality.

For weeks I did not mention these feelings to anyone but my husband. I thought they would pass. I assumed I would come to my senses and miss my breast. I assumed I would get a prosthesis, like most other mastectomy patients, and look, at least to other people, the way I always had. I had been looking forward to getting a real prosthesis ever since the breast care coordinator had showed me one. When she took it out of its box and handed it to me, I couldn't believe my eyes.

It felt almost like a real breast, except that you could hold it in your hands and kind of manipulate it around. I thought about my year as a copywriter for The Sharper Image catalog. Wow, I thought, they could sell a ton of these! When I got home I described it to my husband, who thought it sounded like a fun thing to have around. A close male friend asked if maybe I could get one for him too.

Redefining Normal

As part of her postmastectomy routine, the breast care coordinator at the hospital called Reach To Recovery, the American Cancer Society's volunteer visiting program, to ask that someone visit me. The program sends women who have had breast cancer themselves to visit women newly home from the hospital to offer moral support and a first, temporary prosthesis. Nobody came. I informed the breast care coordinator, and she phoned in her request a second time. Still no response.

I decided to improvise my own temporary prosthesis, and bought a big bag of polyester fiber, the kind used to fill stuffed animals. I carefully stuffed my empty bra cup, arranging and rearranging the fiber, trying to approximate the shape and density of my lost breast. Either I wasn't very good at it or it wasn't such a great idea. The stuffed "breast" kept coming out higher than my real one, and it moved higher still when I walked. After a few days of struggling with it, I discarded the idea, and my bra as well. I took to wearing loose, oversized tee shirts, which were more comfortable anyway in the hot days of late summer.

Feeling fine physically, I eased back into working and gradually forgot to worry about my lopsidedness. Each day it seemed a little bit less important than it had the day before.

After several months, when my chest was completely healed, Dr. S. said I could get myself a real prosthesis. A nurse in the surgery department gave me the names of several stores that specialized in them and told me my health-care plan would cover the cost. I called one of the medical supply stores for information, but I didn't make an appointment for a fitting. I intended to call back when I had more time, but days passed, and then weeks. One thing and then another pushed the prosthesis lower on my list of priorities.

One day, a few months after I called the store, my husband and I were sitting on the patio of our neighborhood cafe, sipping coffee. "You know," I said, "I don't think I'm going to get a prosthesis. I don't really feel the need any more." He wasn't surprised. And by then he didn't care either.

Instead, I bought a sports bra that supports my breast side and lies smoothly over my flat side. I wear it under clothes that are too revealing to wear without any bra. Most days, I don't wear a bra at all. What a free feeling! No elastic or wire cuts into my flesh, no straps dig into my shoulders. I hardly ever think about not being a normally shaped woman, and no one else seems to notice or care. One-breastedness now is normal for me.

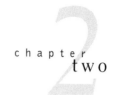
Be Optimistic

(The Odds Are on Your Side)

You may die of breast cancer, but you probably won't.

The fear of breast cancer among American women has reached epidemic proportions. This is not because the number of deaths from
breast cancer is on the rise—that number has changed little in the last
30 years—but rather because breast cancer has moved into the spotlight and is now a public issue. In the past few years, "breast cancer
awareness" has become a common phrase and a political stance. At
high-visibility celebrity functions, pink breast-cancer-awareness lapel
ribbons show up next to red AIDS ribbons. The U.S. Postal Service
issued a breast cancer awareness stamp in 1995, and in 1998 introduced a stamp to raise funds for breast cancer research. Since 1996,
October has been officially designated American Breast Cancer
Awareness Month....

In one way, all of this is good. The more people become concerned
and speak out about a disease, the more money gets put into research
for its cure, and the better the chances a cure, or at least more effective
treatments, will be found. Women have been suffering and dying from
breast cancer for centuries, and it is certainly time for a concerted
effort to conquer it.

On the other hand, the breast cancer "facts" that now appear frequently in the media and in both public and private discussions are distorted in a way that makes me uneasy. The most extreme statistics are
bandied about as if they were the general rule. Negativity and morbid-
ity prevail. In all the talk about breast cancer you rarely hear the fact
that most of the women who get it deal with it and go on to live out
normal, healthy lives. You also rarely hear that fear itself, and a pessimistic attitude, can negatively affect a woman's ability to cope with
the disease.

In pointing out the exaggerations of the breast cancer threat I do
not mean to minimize its importance. There is no question that

advanced breast cancer is a terrifying and deadly disease. Approximately 45,000 American women die from it each year. [3] Their deaths are tragic, and deserving of the attention and concern they are finally getting. Still, it is important to put their experience in perspective. It is important to keep in mind the fact that the vast majority of American women never get breast cancer, and the majority of those who do don't die of it.

The Risk Is Lower Than You Think

During my own breast cancer crisis, I spent a good deal of time trying to untangle the confusing statistics and come to a clear understanding of how the breast cancer "numbers" related to my life and the lives of other women. Like everyone else, I had seen the now well-known "one-in-eight" risk statistic for breast cancer many times. For a long time I simply accepted it as true. I also assumed that those numbers meant one in eight American women would die of breast cancer. I can't say why I assumed that, but I did, and I don't think I'm the only one.

The problem with many statistics is that they are simplified for public consumption, and in the process they get distorted. When I looked into the rather frightening one-in-eight statistic, I found that it doesn't mean at all what it appears to mean. For one thing, the statistic is rarely fully stated. To be complete, it should say that the probability of an American woman being diagnosed with breast cancer *during her lifetime* is one in eight. That may sound like nitpicking, but you cannot understand the numbers until you know what the statisticians mean by "in her lifetime." Most of them define "in her lifetime" in this context as "by the age of 90 or more." An American woman's statistical chance of being diagnosed with breast cancer by the time she is 90 or older has been set at one in eight. [4]

When I discovered the "90 years old" part of the statistic, I thought, well, by the time she's 90 years old a woman's chance of being diagnosed with something serious is going to be pretty damn high anyway. At 90 years old, one in eight doesn't sound that bad. What's more, as I came to understand, those numbers refer only to diagnosis. The death rate from breast cancer is considerably lower. About 70 percent of American women who are diagnosed with breast cancer do not die of it. The statistical chance of dying of breast cancer is about 1 in 26 for a white woman in her lifetime, and 1 in 31 for a black woman.[5] (The risk for Hispanic and Asian women is lower.) So, if you are an American woman and you live to be at least 90 years old, the probability that you'll die of breast cancer is no more than 3.8 percent. There is at least a 96.2 percent chance that you will die of something else. Those numbers I found comforting.

How much chance is there, then, that an average American woman will get breast cancer? The most frequently quoted statistics show that the chance that a woman will be diagnosed by age 30 is 1 in 2500, or 0.04 percent. That means that out of every 2500 women up to age 30, only one would be expected to be diagnosed. The chance of being diagnosed by age 40 is 1 in 217, less than one-half of one percent. By age 50 the probability jumps to 1 in 50, or 2 percent, still a fairly modest number. By age 70 the risk is set at 1 in 14, or 7.14 percent, and by age 80 (the current life expectancy for American women), it's 1 in 10, or 10 percent.[6] (I was surprised to learn that men, too, can get breast cancer—approximately 1 in 100 cases is a man.)

As I struggled to understand how statistics in general work, what information they clarify, and what they obscure, a friend of a friend, someone who actually understands statistics, spent a frustrating hour trying to help me to see the light. One of the things he pointed out was that since the risk statistics for breast cancer are expressed as "by the age of," as a woman gets older her risk actually goes down, because she has already passed through some of the statistical categories unscathed. For instance, the risk of being diagnosed with breast cancer by age 90 is one in eight, or 12.5 women per 100, and the risk of being diagnosed by age 70 is 1 in 14, or 7.14 per hundred. If you are 70 and don't have breast cancer, what is your chance of being diagnosed by the time you are 90? According to the statistics, at least 7 of 100 women have already been diagnosed with breast cancer by age 70, and you are not one of them. That means only 5 more per 100 will be diagnosed in your age group in the next 20 years. Your chance of being one of them is therefore 1 in 20. By the same formula, if you are 50 and don't have the disease, your chance of being diagnosed by age 70 is also about 1 in 20. Of the approximately seven women who will be diagnosed by age 70, two have already been diagnosed by age 50. That leaves 5 per 100 to be diagnosed over the next 20 years.

This leads to a good example of how statistics get manipulated. The longer the time frame you look at, the worse the risk statistics appear. Although the breast cancer risk between ages 50 and 70 is about 1 in 20, and the risk from age 70 to age 90 is also 1 in 20, if you look at the entire 40-year period from age 50 to age 90, you get to compound the risk and you come up with 1 in 10. People who want the situation to appear as frightening as possible look at as long a time span as possible. [7]

Taken by themselves, all of these numbers are just generalizations. To make them apply to you, you have to consider all the factors that are currently thought to affect the risk for an individual woman. (With all due respect, I am leaving the rare male cases out of this discussion.) Besides age, these are family history, smoking, exposure to pollution and various environmental poisons, at what age you began menstruating, whether and when you have given birth, whether and when you breast-fed, whether you have passed menopause, whether you are taking or have taken estrogen, whether you exercise regularly, your diet, how much stress you experience ... the list of possible contributing or extenuating factors is so long and so difficult to evaluate that the attempt quickly becomes an exercise in frustration.

Even the factors we think are obvious become slippery when you examine them closely. Take the fact that a woman is more likely to develop breast cancer if her mother or sister had it. That is indeed true; it is borne out by the statistics, and women who do not have a family history of breast cancer surely find comfort in it. However, look a little deeper and you find that the risk is significantly higher only if the mother or sister developed the cancer before menopause. Postmenopausal breast cancer does not appear to be hereditary. What's more—and this I was amazed to discover—nearly 95 percent of women who are diagnosed with breast cancer are *not* daughters or sisters of former breast cancer patients. [8] So while it is true that heredity puts some women at greater risk, it doesn't do much to protect the rest.

I emerged from my investigation of breast cancer statistics with the firm conviction that it's best to leave the numbers to the experts, who seem to enjoy them. Statistics are too convoluted, too difficult to understand, and too easy to manipulate in one direction or another for them to be of much use to the average woman. What I want to know is simple. Is my cancer likely to return? Will breast cancer strike my friends? Or my daughter? But life is not simple; it refuses to be quantified. The answer to each of my questions is, nobody knows.

What did become obvious through my battle with statistics is that there is no cause for breast cancer panic, no need for American women to walk around feeling that the threat of breast cancer is hanging over our heads like the sword of Damocles. We would all be better off putting our energies into enjoying our lives rather than fearing our potential demise. The bottom line is this: even if we live to be 90 years old or older (one source actually set 110 as the "lifetime" measure) [9], nearly 88 percent of us will not have to deal with breast cancer. Even if we live to be 90 years old or older, some 96 percent of us will die of something else.

All this doesn't change the fact that many of us will find potentially dangerous lumps in our breasts. If we are smart we will be on the lookout, examining our breasts regularly, and will have mammograms at once to check out any lumps we find. Being less fearful doesn't mean being less vigilant. In most cases a lump will prove to be harmless. To call up yet another statistic, about 95 percent of abnormalities that show up on mammograms turn out, after further testing, not to be cancer. [10]

On the other hand, it is important to remember that mammograms are not infallible; they do not catch all cancerous breast lumps. While the chances of having breast cancer are small, they are real, and it can be dangerous to depend too heavily on any one test. Every woman needs to be aware of changes in her breast. If you feel something is wrong, regardless of what a mammogram shows, you should pursue further tests.

Fear, Too, Is a Disease

❋

I think it is important to ask whether by exaggerating the risk and the destructiveness of breast cancer, those who are campaigning for more attention and more research for the disease stir up unhealthy and unnecessary levels of fear, and by doing so are inadvertently hurting the women they are trying to help. We have all heard breast cancer called "a woman's worst nightmare." I believe, having been there, that the breast cancer nightmare is the fear, negativity, and pessimism that surround the disease, making it harder for those who get it to deal with it, and haunting even those who will never get it.

The fear of breast cancer has skyrocketed in recent years, despite the fact that the number of annual deaths from the disease has stayed essentially the same for decades. Given the fact that the number of diagnoses has gone up as diagnostic tests have improved, the death rate from breast cancer has actually gone down. Nor is breast cancer the rampant killer that many people think it is.[11] More American women actually die each year from lung cancer. According to official reports, lung cancer kills some 56,000 American women each year, nearly 25 percent more than breast cancer. Even that number pales next to the figures for the greatest threat to American women, heart disease, which kills approximately 500,000 women each year—more than eleven times as many as die from breast cancer.

One of the major reasons so many women think of breast cancer as a death sentence is that doctors are extremely cautious in what they say to and about their breast cancer patients. Most doctors will tell you that regardless of how small a breast tumor is, or how early it is caught, it is impossible to know for certain that it has not sent out microscopic cancer cells that are capable of growing elsewhere in the body. Since they still don't have any way of knowing for certain that a cancer has not spread, and they don't know how to predict who might have a recurrence, they simply don't talk about anybody being cured. They refer instead to patients who have been "cancer-free" for a given number of years, making it sound like every one of us is teetering on the brink, just moments away from a relapse.

Well, my mother, who had a mastectomy in her late 50s, has been "cancer-free" for nearly 30 years. By the authority vested in me as a sensible, logical person, I hereby declare her cured. The same goes for my friend Henry's mother, and my friend Sandy's mother. There are millions of women who have been walking around "cancer-free" for as many as 20, 30, or 40 years. Some of them may face cancer again, but most of them, as far as I am concerned, are cured.

I expect some women will think me disrespectful for suggesting this, but I think it is time we turn some of our focus from the losers in the fight against breast cancer to the winners. I do not belittle in any way the pain or tragedy of those who have succumbed. Their story is powerful and immensely important. But it is only part of the story, and the smaller part at that. Our preoccupation with those who die of breast cancer has kept us from being encouraged and inspired by the many more who live—long and well.

chapter three

Take Your Time, But Not Too Much

There is enough time.

When you are diagnosed with a serious illness, time becomes something you worry about. *How much do I have left?* you wonder franti-
cally. *How much can I take to decide what I should do? How much difference will it make in the long run if I rush too quickly to a decision,
or wait too long to take action?...*

I was surprised that Dr. R., while telling me the two lumps in my
breast were malignant, also said I had time to think about what I wanted to do. I remembered that when my mother had her biopsy, she was
kept under anesthesia while the hospital lab ran its tests. They determined that her tumor was malignant and her surgeon removed her
entire breast, as well as the muscles behind it, without giving her a
chance to decide anything.

Since then, researchers have concluded that breast cancer, once
thought to grow and spread quickly, actually grows relatively slowly.
The generally accepted scenario is that breast cancer starts with a single cell, which takes approximately 100 days to double to two cells.
The two-cell structure takes approximately another 100 days to double
to four cells. And another 100 days to double to eight. Every hundred
days the number of cells doubles. [12]

Cells being the tiny things they are, it takes quite a while before a
breast cancer has grown big enough to be felt, or even detected on a
mammogram. A 1-centimeter breast tumor, about the smallest size
you can feel with your fingers, contains some 100 billion cells and has
most likely been growing for a good 10 years. A tumor that is too small
to feel but shows up on a mammogram may have been growing for as
long as 9 years and probably contains about 10 billion cells.

I sat down with a pencil and paper one day and calculated the number of cells at each 100 days. I broke my columns of figures with horizontal lines that indicated the passage of years. I am not usually swept
up by math, but this exercise was dramatic. At first the totals looked

insignificant, not much to worry about. According to the formula, after about a year a new cancer has only eight cells. After two years, it has only 128. Then the numbers start to jump. In three years, there are more than 2,000 cells; in four years, more than 16,000. It really became unnerving when I got to the seven-year mark—more than 33 million cells. At slightly past eight years the count hit a billion.

I came away from my little math exercise shaken and sobered. I had been relieved, after my biopsy, to be told that taking a few weeks to gather my energies and make a decision about mastectomy wasn't likely to make much difference in my prospects. After seeing the numbers on paper, I was even more relieved that I hadn't waited any longer. The two weeks Dr. R. gave me to think, research, get a second opinion if I wanted one, and generally acclimate myself to the idea that I had cancer was a perfect length of time. It was long enough to gather my thoughts and a lot of information, but not so long that I could avoid the subject. In all, it was about two months from the night I found my lumps to the day of my biopsy, which removed them.[13] Each measured about 1.5 centimeters in diameter. About one month later my mastectomy removed all remaining traces of malignancy and proved my lymph nodes to be unaffected.

Move Carefully, But Keep Moving

Once you realize how quickly the size of a tumor increases, you see how important it is for any woman who finds a breast lump to take immediate action. And yet, many delay. Sometimes it is because they are overwhelmed by their own doubts or fears. Sometimes it is because their doctors elect to take a wait-and-see approach after feeling a lump. The latter is inexplicable to me. I can understand a woman being paralyzed by her fear or, given the many public misconceptions about breast cancer, simply not knowing how much difference immediate action can make. Doctors, on the other hand, should know better. If they err, it should be on the side of caution. My own doctors, although they really seemed to believe my lumps would turn out not to be malignant, kept sending me from test to test, determined to find out for sure. I will always be grateful to them. Because of their persistence I, too, kept pursuing an answer, and as a result dealt with my tumors while they were still small and, apparently, had not yet spread.

I was upset when a young friend recently told me about her step-mother's experience. Her doctor felt a lump in her breast but instead of taking action he recommended watching it for a year. While he "watched," her cancer grew. Since it was initially large enough to feel, it was probably at about the ten-year, one-centimeter stage, and had approximately 100 billion cells. A year later it must have been in the range of two centimeters and had more than a trillion cells! The doctor finally took action and my friend's stepmother had a mastectomy, which had to be followed by both radiation and chemotherapy. I cannot help wondering if she could have avoided those powerful, invasive follow-up treatments if her doctor had been more aggressive a year earlier.

Why are some doctors slow to take action when they find breast lumps? I think one major reason is that breast lumps are extremely common, and most of them turn out to be harmless. Some women have naturally lumpy breasts, with lumps that come and go with every menstrual cycle. Other women, with relatively smooth breasts, find three or four lumps in a lifetime, all of which turn out to be no threat to their health.

Doctors are aware of the statistics. They know that chances are good a lump will turn out not to be cancer, especially if it is in the breast of a woman who has had similar lumps in the past. [14] The problem, of course, is that any woman at any time, whether she has had harmless breast lumps in the past or not, can suddenly develop a lump that is cancer, and that can turn fatal if it is not treated early enough.

You Can Learn a Lot by Talking

Before my own cancer experience, I didn't realize how common it is for women to find lumps in their breasts. I found out because I am by nature a talker, a starter of conversations. As I pushed on through my seemingly endless tests, I felt a strong need to talk to other women about my situation. I'm not sure what I was looking for—support, I guess, and sympathy too. I found both, and far more camaraderie than I ever expected. Some days it seemed as if every woman I talked to had had a biopsy herself or had been called back for further examination after a routine mammogram. I was amazed. None of these women had ever mentioned their experiences to me before. Once I broached the subject, the stories, and the worries, came tumbling out.

One good friend took me into her bedroom and lifted her shirt to show me her biopsy scar. Why hadn't she mentioned anything to me when she was going through the trauma of thinking she might have cancer? She said she had wanted to, but just never found a way to bring the subject up. Her husband had given her good support, she said, but it would have helped to have a woman friend to talk to. When her lump had proved to be harmless, she had pushed the whole experience out of her mind.

Three other friends I mentioned my situation to during those first emotional weeks responded to my story with their own. One said she had fibrous breasts and was always finding worrisome lumps. The other two were both waiting for laboratory test results. Neither turned out to have cancer.

Even as I was enjoying the genuine understanding and empathy of these women friends, I was disturbed by the fact that they had not told me about their experiences before. Each of them had chosen to suffer in terrified silence while waiting for news from the pathology lab, then each dismissed her experience when her lump turned out not to be cancer. As a friend, I wished they had given me the opportunity to offer my support; as a woman facing my own diagnosis, I was upset that they had not shared what they knew. They had the kind of information I was looking for; they had experienced the kinds of tests and consultations that loomed before me. There I was starting from scratch, searching for information to guide me, looking for encouragement, and everyone I knew who had been through the same struggle was silent until I began to talk.

Would it really make a difference if women talked to each other about our breast cancer scares? You bet it would. When you find yourself caught in a frightening situation in which making the best decision quickly can be a major factor in your prospects for survival, every bit of shared information is valuable.

Perhaps even more importantly, if we share our experiences as they occur, more women will know what it's like to face the possibility of breast cancer *before* they ever have to experience it themselves. If we all help our friends through their testing ordeals, and see most of them turn out to be false alarms, we will be less frightened if we find a lump ourselves, and more likely to take speedy action. Having seen other women cope with the same situation, we will know what to expect. We will know if a doctor is taking our lump more casually than he or she should, possibly endangering our lives by choosing to wait and see what develops. We will say to ourselves, *My friend's doctor kept testing until she knew for sure. I want mine to do the same.*

With all the attention that is now focused on breast cancer, why does a woman have to wait until she is diagnosed with a malignancy to have a support group she can turn to? It is a question that bothers me deeply, and I don't have an answer. Do we hesitate to speak to each other because we have been taught that health matters are private? Did our teenage experiences saddle us with a self-consciousness about our breasts that we have never been able to shake off? Are we perhaps afraid that people will shy away from us if they think we are ill? Whatever our reasons, by not talking about our breast cancer fears and experiences we are doing ourselves and each other a massive disservice, both physically and psychologically.

Luckily, the four friends I have referred to all took immediate medical action. They saw a physical threat to their health and took steps to protect themselves. But they still suffered unnecessarily because they considered the psychological and emotional blows they endured to be a separate issue, something they could neither share nor do much to protect themselves from, something they just had to bear.

One of the lessons I learned from my own breast cancer experience is that the emotional/psychological impact of a disease like breast cancer is inextricably intertwined with its physical aspects. Inevitably, with the threat of breast cancer comes fear, and fear is a powerful and destructive force that takes a toll on the body as well as the mind. In fact, since breast cancer in its early stages does not cause physical pain or discomfort, from the moment of discovering a breast lump, fear and emotional turmoil are the major symptoms most women have to deal with.

The most tragic cases are those women who discover a lump in a breast and are so paralyzed by their fear they don't tell anyone, and don't seek medical help. Those women, I hope, are a small minority, but even among the women who do seek medical advice and treatment, there are way too many who suffer because they can't bring themselves to talk openly about breast cancer with family and friends. Forced to deal with their anxieties alone, some find a false and dangerous comfort in denial. In the course of doing research for this book I came across a fascinating study conducted in the 1970s by a Swedish psychologist named Karin Gyllensköld. [15] Trying to understand the psychological impact of breast cancer, she interviewed women just after they had received a breast cancer diagnosis and several times more as they progressed through treatment. It is disturbing to read excerpts from interviews in which some of the women admit that right up to the time of their surgery they had convinced themselves the doctors had made a mistake, or the hospital had mixed up their records. They kept expecting the mistake to be discovered and the cancer to be gone. Such denial, and the isolation it feeds on, are all-too-common consequences of our allowing our fears to cut us off from one another.

The Mind-Body Disconnection

I sometimes wish that breast cancer were a painful disease right from the start. That way it would be difficult to ignore or deny. The fact that for most women breast cancer causes no pain is what makes it especially insidious. Because time is so vital, it is important to take seriously the possibility that any breast lump may mean cancer, and yet it is so hard to believe you may be ill, even deathly ill, when you are feeling absolutely fine. We learn from early childhood that our bodies know when something is wrong and quickly tell us. The smallest cut or scrape causes pain. A splinter so small you can't see it without a magnifying glass pricks incessantly until you manage to get it out. With breast cancer, you get up in the morning feeling full of energy and good health, and you ask yourself, do I really want to go on slogging through the tests and consultations that may simply prove nothing is wrong with me?

Even after my postbiopsy consultation, as I sat in the hospital breast care coordinator's office with a copy of my pathology report in my hand, my mind turned away, refusing to believe. I felt as though I were reading about somebody else. How could a report written by a technician in some distant lab prove that I had cancer when my own body wasn't giving me the slightest hint that something was wrong? You hear a lot these days about the importance of the mind-body connection. This was a total mind-body disconnection. I knew I had to believe that I had breast cancer, and yet I couldn't believe it.

I lost count of how many times I read that pathology report. For days it sat on my desk as I tried to work, constantly distracting me from the task at hand. Each time I read it, it felt a bit more familiar, but I never was able to connect the danger it reported to any feeling in my chest. In the end I simply had to tell myself it was true and there was no point in denying it. I have never felt so alienated from my own body, or felt so desperate to find a way to pull the parts of myself together.

After Diagnosis, Stop and Think

I think every woman with breast cancer comes to a crossroad, a place where she has to choose the path she is going to take. If you are moving too fast, or are too caught up in your emotions, it is possible not to notice. You can race right on through, oblivious to the fact that other roads, perhaps less traveled than the one you are on, are branching off in different directions. It is important to slow down, to look around, to think before you choose which way to go.

I am not referring to the wrenching decisions of which treatments to choose. Before you can tackle those terribly important choices, there is an even more important, much more basic decision to be made. You must decide how you, a woman who has just received a diagnosis of breast cancer, are going to live your life from this day on. Here at the place where you know at last that you have cancer, you need to stop and gather yourself together. Here is where you force yourself to set aside the feeling of urgency that has driven you through all the tests. Here you give yourself a little time.

A diagnosis of cancer brings on a collision with reality. This is it. Life and death. The impact is tremendous and sends you reeling. Beneath the racing emotions and the raging fear there is a numbing feeling of bewilderment, a sense of aloneness in a world of decisions you don't have any idea how to make.

Most of us go through life without looking very carefully at ourselves. We move from day to day, from job to job, from relationship to relationship without ever asking ourselves the big questions: *What do I really care about? What do I fear? What kind of sacrifices am I willing to make and what kind of risks am I willing to take to get what I really want? And just what is it that I really want?* We let our lives be shaped pretty much from the outside, by our jobs, our friends, our church, our community. We wear the same clothes, watch the same movies and television programs, listen to the same authorities, and internalize the same myths as everyone around us. It takes a crisis to make us stop and think.

During the two weeks between my cancer diagnosis and the dead-line I had accepted for deciding how to proceed, I spent a lot of time trying to figure myself out. I tried desperately to bring deep feelings to the surface where I could know them. I stared at my left breast and tried to feel the emotions stirred by the thought of losing it. I looked at my husband and my daughter and tried to feel my love for them phys-ically, in my body. I measured the emotions I was pushing myself to feel against the assumptions I had about my life, trying to decide which ones fit together and which didn't.

As I sorted out my feelings, some of the assumptions I had unthinkingly accepted about my body and my life began to fall away. I grew certain that saving my breast wasn't important to me and that surgery was something I could handle, but I also realized how afraid I was of being sick and of the pressures my being sick would put on my relationships.

Little by little, I began to see how I wanted to proceed. The main thing I decided was that I would not let cancer take over my life. I knew if I decided I was sick I could make myself feel sick; my mind had that power. Instead I decided to concentrate on continuing to feel fine. Maybe in the end cancer would get me and I would die, but for as long as I could, I would do everything possible to extend and enjoy my life.

I think the upbeat tone I deliberately set changed my entire approach to my illness and was, in fact, my first step toward healing. The positive picture of myself that came into focus kept me on a course I felt comfortable with, despite some powerful pressures, through my mastectomy and the months that followed, as I made my way back to health.

As I look back, I am glad that I pushed hard and persevered through the early months of testing, until I reached a definite diagnosis. And I am equally glad that once I knew what was going on in my body, I paused long enough to make my own diagnosis of what was going on in my mind, my heart, and my life. I would urge any woman facing the enormous challenges of breast cancer to do the same.

Avoid the Worry Trap

*Worry makes
things worse.*

I am an accomplished worrier. I am good at it because I get so much practice. I worry about big things and ridiculously insignificant things. I lie awake at night worrying about everything from being able to pay this month's bills to whether the public library will cut me off for keeping a book two days too long. I worry that a friend may have misinterpreted a comment I made; that the UPS truck will come as soon as I go into the bathroom; that my daughter will be mad at me for sending her to school without an umbrella on a day it wasn't supposed to rain, but did. I know how silly it is to worry about things you cannot control, and I know how hard it is to stop....

Worrying is one of the most destructive things you can do to yourself. Not only does it weaken you by robbing you of sleep and making you tense and nervous, it actually enables whatever it is you're worried about to feed on your strength and grow. Small problems grow into giants when you worry about them. Big problems become all-consuming.

It would be foolish for me to say that a woman who discovers a suspicious lump in her breast shouldn't worry about it. Or that a woman whose biopsy proves her lump to be malignant should expect to sit down calmly and coolly to plan out what to do. If you think you might have breast cancer, you are going to worry. If you find out for certain that you have it, you are going to worry big. None of us can banish worry altogether. But if we see worry for the destructive force it is, we can do something about controlling it.

Keeping It All in Perspective

❀

I believe I have found an antidote to worry. It is perspective. When a threat is looming in your life, it is very important to keep it in perspective, to look at it in relation to all that surrounds it. Things that appear huge when we focus in on them can shrink considerably when we pull back and take a broader view.

We have all seen movie monsters that appear as large as tall buildings, lumbering along crushing cars and houses as if they were matchsticks. Occasionally we get to see a documentary on how a monster film was made. We see the "monster" in the studio and realize it is only a foot tall. The houses and cars its mechanical step crushes are tiny models on a table, designed to collapse easily. That is not to say that all monsters are optical illusions. There are real-life threats in the world, and some of them truly are big and dangerous. The point is simply that it is hard to know how big a threat really is until you can see the whole picture.

An advanced, aggressive cancer is an honest-to-goodness monster, capable of crushing a life. But most breast cancers are much smaller and can be effectively treated. More importantly, most breast lumps are not cancer at all. One day perhaps there will be a quick way to diagnose breast cancer, and a woman who finds a lump in her breast will know in a matter of days, or even hours, if she is facing a real threat, a temporary health problem, or a false alarm. For now, unfortunately, it often takes many tests over the course of several weeks to determine whether a lump is malignant and, if so, how big and how serious it is. Getting through the days of not knowing without letting worry eat you alive can be a major challenge.

Human nature is such that even though we know most breast lumps do not turn out to be cancer, every woman worries that hers is the real thing. From the very first sign that something may be wrong, we all can benefit from a dose of perspective. If you find a lump in your breast, or something suspicious turns up on a mammogram, the best thing you can do for yourself is take a deep breath and pull your mind back until you can see the full stage on which this particular monster looms. Remind yourself that millions of lumps show up on mammograms and during routine breast exams, of which yours is just one. You aren't suddenly tumbling to your doom. You're going through a normal female event, not a pleasant event, but not an unusual one either. You have to do what women do in these circumstances, which is to be tested and find out what's going on. While you're waiting for the answer, if you let yourself jump to negative conclusions you may start your whole life unraveling.

The best thing to do while you wait is to carry on with whatever you were doing before the lump popped up. It could be a month or more before you know enough to take action. That waiting time is a chunk of your life; like every other time in your life, it can be as full or as empty as you decide to make it. Regardless of what you do while you're waiting, the result of your tests will be the same. You cannot change the outcome by worrying. All worrying does is make you miserable.

If you're like most women, one or two tests will be the full extent of your breast cancer experience. Your lump will turn out to be a cyst or a benign tumor or some other irregularity that is no threat to your health. You'll heave a sigh of relief and go back to things as they were.

But what if your early tests produce inconclusive results or flat-out bad news? Then you will be facing more tests, more waiting, and more challenges to keeping your imagination and your fears under control. You'd best understand from the outset that worry is an opportunist; it will jump in to fill any empty spaces in your life. The best way to prevent it from seizing control is to accept that there is no way to know what the future may hold, and to focus on living in the present.

You'll probably find, as I did, that the medical tests for breast cancer are not hard to deal with. The mammogram, which squeezed my breast flat between two glass plates, was the most uncomfortable, but none of the tests I had was painful and, until I got to a surgical biopsy, each took only a few minutes. The problems were all psychological, and they stemmed from waiting for results, not the tests themselves. Hungry for answers, I tried at every stage to wheedle information from whoever was doing the test of the moment. I got nowhere and finally had to give in to the protocol that keeps medical technicians from speculating on the results of their tests. Though I hated it, I can see why it is that way. No one wants to give out information that may later turn out to be wrong. And, in our very litigious society, no one wants to take a chance of being sued. So don't expect to get quick or unofficial answers. You'll only be setting yourself up for frustration, and there's enough of that without your adding to it.

Staying Whole When Your World Is Split in Two
❧

When you go through a battery of medical tests, you learn pretty fast that being a patient means having to be patient. It may not be your normal way of reacting to the world. It certainly wasn't mine. You eventually come to realize that our modern health-care institutions run on their own schedule, and nothing you can do will speed it up. What's more, they function in their own separate, strange version of reality.

This fact of two simultaneous realities dawned on me one day as I was driving home from another test at the hospital. I suddenly saw that I was living my life in two separate worlds, and I was actually acting like two different people. Each time I walked into the hospital, I became a patient, someone who was there to be probed and photographed, pricked and palpated. I was someone who was expected to dress and undress on command, sit half-naked in a tiny room waiting for a polite knock on the door, and turn over the care of my body to a stranger who was trained to understand what was happening to it better than I did. Something about the atmosphere of the hospital was able to transform me on each visit from a strong, self-confident adult into an obedient child.

My whole demeanor changed when I walked into the hospital. I became compliant, mostly silent, reluctant to speak up for myself or to complain. I was the passive receiver of tests, instructions, and evaluations. I was someone I hardly knew. After a half hour in this almost surreal environment, I would put my clothes back on and step out into the sunshine. Instantly I was the old familiar me again, walking with a determined stride back to my car.

I noticed on that particular day that I had developed a routine. As I had a number of times before, as soon as I got back in my car I pushed a favorite rock 'n' roll cassette into the tape player. I had actually set it out on the seat before walking to the hospital so that when I got back it would be ready to go. I started it playing before I even turned on the engine. I leaned back for a few moments as the car and my mind filled with music. Then I turned the volume up a few notches so I could feel the familiar, powerful beat pulsing in my body, physically pulling me back into the world where I decide who to listen to, where I'm the one who pushes the buttons and turns the dials.

The Power of Rituals

It struck me that the car, the tape player, the well-loved music were vehicles that carried me back into a setting where I felt I had control, away from a deeply disturbing one where I felt I had none. Without consciously thinking about it, I had developed a ritual that transported me quickly from the unpleasant medical part of my life to the comfortable nonmedical part. I was impressed with the way my instincts had worked to ease my stress, or at least limit its sphere of influence. As I thought about it, I saw that I had coped with other stressful situations similarly in the past.

Several times in my life I have held jobs that required me to spend eight hours a day in a San Francisco office building, which, like a hospital, is a setting in which I feel too regimented and restricted to be comfortable. I lived on the other side of San Francisco Bay and always commuted by bus, over a bridge clogged with traffic, even though taking the subway under the bay would have been quicker. Crossing the bridge was an important ritual for me. As the bus rolled slowly eastward at the end of the day, I could feel myself unwinding, relaxing; it was almost as if I was reentering my body after being forced for hours to occupy somebody else's. By the time I reached my stop the pressures and frustrations of the job had melted away.

In many ways my time at the hospital wasn't all that different from my time on the job. In both situations I had to show up at the designated time and place and submit to other people's routines. I had to acknowledge that while I was there someone else was in charge. When forced by financial necessity to work in an office setting, I had developed a ritual that kept the two parts of my life separate and carried me safely from one to the other. When I was forced by medical necessity to submit to testing at the hospital, I had unconsciously developed a similar ritual.

We tend to think of rituals in the context of religious ceremonies or other symbolic events. In truth, we all partake of rituals in our everyday lives. They are powerful tools for creating moods and a sense of self. You probably have rituals you are already using, without even realizing it, to move yourself out of one state of mind and into another. By deliberately scheduling them before or after your doctors' appointments, you can use them to confine your medical experience to just the time it actually requires.

Think about what you do to calm yourself when you're upset or give yourself a relaxing break when life gets too hectic. A cup of tea perhaps, a bubble bath, a walk in a favorite place. Think about the things you have or do that make you feel strong, balanced, and in charge of your life. It may be listening to your favorite music, wearing a favorite piece of jewelry or a hat you particularly like, going for a run, a swim, or an aerobic workout. Doing whatever makes you feel most like you—wearing that hat to your appointment or lounging in that bath immediately afterward—can become the private ritual that quickly carries you back into your own world after each trip to the doctor's office or hospital.

It is a trick of the mind that is well worth playing on yourself. If you don't find a way to keep your medical concerns confined to their proper place, they will slop over into the rest of your life and change the whole tone of your existence. The truth is that you probably won't be able to completely keep your medical ordeal from dragging you down. I know I didn't succeed completely, but I was able to reduce its power over me significantly.

When All Else Fails, Try Distraction

There were days when it was hard to keep worry away. That's when I depended on another powerful weapon—distraction. I tried various things but soon discovered that for me the only distractions that worked were those that filled my mind with sound, and not just any sound, but specifically human voices. I know quiet activities like cooking, jogging, doing a crafts project, or reading a good mystery keep other people engrossed for hours. They don't work for me. There's a part of my mind that is not engaged by those activities. It seizes on the opportunity to take off on its own, exploring the very thoughts I'm trying to avoid. So during those weeks of waiting for test results, I spent more than my usual amount of time talking to friends. Not only did the conversations give me an opportunity to explore my feelings, they occupied my mind when it needed to be occupied and boosted my spirits. The telephone was my great ally. So was my CD player. When I felt down and didn't want to talk, I listened to music, loud music with lyrics. Even just a few minutes with a favorite album always managed to brighten my day and improve my mood.

If you are waiting for test results and you want to keep worry from driving you crazy, it's up to you to find the perspectives and distractions that work for you. This may sound strange, but the search can actually become a fascinating and positive sidelight to your breast cancer experience. You will not only find activities to help you get through the waiting, you will learn some interesting things about how your own mind works.

You may think me a cockeyed optimist, but I believe there is potential for something positive in just about any experience, although we often don't recognize it or take advantage of it. I know I'm not the only woman who feels she benefited from her encounter with breast cancer. Many women who have gone through a scare, or breast cancer itself, say they learned about themselves in the process, and that made their lives better afterwards. If you cannot avoid the experience, you may as well use it in your favor. Instead of letting yourself be swept along by the fear, the worry, the feelings of helplessness that can accompany any major illness, you can take control of your situation, set your own boundaries, and find the keys to inner strength that will not only get you through, but will help you deal with future challenges, both health-related and others as well.

Even with Cancer, You're Still You

For me, all the tests and waiting led finally to the big, final test, a surgical biopsy. I was told that my lumps would be removed in the procedure, so even if they proved to be malignant, my problem would already be solved. It was a simple, outpatient surgery, and I went into it believing that whatever the results, this would be the last step.

On the day of my follow-up consultation, I felt calm and confident. Certain that my ordeal was over, I went alone. I was not in any way prepared for what Dr. R. had to say. In truth, he seemed surprised himself by the pathology report. I was in shock. Instead of the clean bill of health I felt I had been promised, I got a recommendation of mastectomy. Instead of walking out of the hospital cured, I walked out a full-fledged cancer patient. During the long testing period I had found it possible, if not easy, to keep my medical worries on the periphery of my life. Now I was a bona fide cancer patient, and I couldn't keep the tone of my life from changing.

As soon as the diagnosis of cancer is certain, everyone you know focuses their attention on your health. That doesn't mean other aspects of your life disappear. You are still a wife, a mother, a friend, a computer programmer, a teacher, whatever you were before, but those roles seem to fade temporarily. It's as if each aspect of your life is an actor in a play, and suddenly the actor playing health takes center stage to deliver an emotional speech. The spotlight focuses in, and all the other members of the cast are left in shadow. They're still there, moving around, speaking softly, but it's hard for anyone to see them or hear them. For as long as the monologue lasts, health dominates the stage.

It is easy to lose sight of the fact that cancer is only one of the many things that are going on in your life. I had to keep reminding myself and everyone else who was close to me that, as intense as it was, this time would pass. One way or another I would come out on the other side of cancer treatment. Of course, I had no way of predicting whether a return to health or a sadly shortened life lay ahead for me. I was worried, but at the same time I knew I couldn't live day after day with the intense emotions that come with that kind of worry. So I began looking for a way to turn it off.

The obvious answer was to increase my emphasis on living in the present. Whether I was going to live or die in the long run, I was very much alive for the moment, and was feeling fine besides. If my condition was going to get serious, there would be plenty of time for suffering later. A reality check turned up some powerful arguments in my favor. Although sometimes it seemed to me that the biopsy report had changed everything in my life, nothing had really changed at all. I wasn't in pain or feeling especially tired. In fact, I wasn't incapacitated in any way. The only changes that had taken place were in my mind, where worry, fear, and imagined scenes of my impending death had temporarily taken an upper hand. It was true that there would be more visits to the hospital now, and a major surgery, but none of that was going to take up very much time. My health problems had moved to a more serious level, but they were still confined to a limited portion of my life.

When some people discover they have cancer, they let all their other concerns and responsibilities, and even their relationships, start to slide. I understand how that can happen. There are times when you feel frustrated, angry, and very sorry for yourself. If you don't guard against it, it's easy to get depressed and sink into despair, convinced that your life is about to end, tragically and prematurely. Why go on? It's cancer. Why not just give up?

As I thought about it, I came up with lots of reasons. The one that did most to keep me going was knowing that I just might survive. After all, most women who get breast cancer do. I asked myself, *What's going to happen if you don't keep your life going? If you stop seeing friends and turn down new projects?* The answer was obvious. Suddenly the treatment would be over and I'd be anxious to get back to my normal life. Would it still be there? I figured I'd better keep things going.

Assertiveness Is Good for the Soul
❀

After my diagnosis I gave myself a few days to feel really awful about my situation, then I said enough of that. It can be hard to keep social activities going when you're worried about dying, but for me it felt even harder to go through day after day carrying my concerns alone. It's a question of what kind of energy you want suffusing your life. To be sociable you have to summon up positive, upbeat energy. You have to allow yourself to relax, let your hair down a little, laugh, and appreciate the warmth of others. It seems to me that positive energy is the best kind to have flowing through you in difficult times.

As luck would have it, my cancer diagnosis came about two and a half weeks before I was scheduled to go to Hawaii with my husband and daughter. For as long as I could remember I had dreamed of a Hawaiian vacation, but had never managed to get there. Then my husband was invited to a conference on Maui and we decided finally to do it. The tickets were bought and the condo by the beach reserved when the damned biopsy came back positive and threatened to ruin it all.

My appointment for a second opinion was on July 10, just a week before our planned trip. I was agonizing over whether or not to go, but I hadn't cancelled any reservations. When Dr. S. confirmed my diagnosis, he urged me to schedule surgery right away. I asked if he would perform the operation, and he went to his office to get his calendar. When he walked back into the examining room, I took a deep breath and said, as calmly as I could, that I was going to Hawaii for a week and would like to schedule the operation for after my return. I watched his face, afraid I was in for a lecture about the gravity of my situation. He flipped the page of his appointment book. "When will you be back?" he asked.

To my surprise, he thought a vacation just before surgery was a great idea. My gynecologist, with whom I had a consultation the next day, thought so too. So ten days before my mastectomy I took off with my family for the beaches and sunshine of Maui. Talk about ways to drive worry out of your mind!

The beach was a five-minute walk from our room; it was uncrowded and unbelievably beautiful. The colors and patterns on the tropical fish, which swam in close to shore, were exquisite. Even the rain, when it fell one afternoon, was warm and friendly. I loved Hawaii. My 9-year-old daughter, whose swimming had been a bit tentative before, grew suddenly bold in this gentle environment. She put on flippers and a face mask and swam out well over her head to float with my husband and me on the surface of the water and gaze down at the fish swimming below. Never had the three of us felt closer, or happier. Between Jay's conference meetings, we explored the island, ate marvelous meals, hiked into the crater of the Haleakala volcano, attended an unabashedly touristy luau, bought muumuus and Hawaiian print shirts, and generally had the time of our lives. Day after day I forgot to think about cancer and my upcoming surgery. When thoughts of what awaited me at home crept into my mind at night, just before sleep, they seemed distant and not terribly threatening. It's hard to think morbid thoughts when you're living a dream.

I came back to California relaxed, tanned, and ready to face anything. The next day I walked into the hospital for pre-operation tests feeling healthy, centered, and strong. I had just had one of the best weeks of my life, and I had given it to myself. I had not cancelled my vacation plans. I had asserted myself and made the people at the hospital fit their schedule to mine, and I'd found out, to my surprise, that that was fine with them. I suddenly felt less like a pawn and more like a participant in this medical journey I was on. Having taken some control over what was happening to me, I felt more comfortable conceding the rest to others. I was looking forward to having my surgery and moving beyond it. The people who surrounded me in the hospital seemed anxious to help me get through whatever lay ahead. They were on my side.

The funny thing is that no one at the hospital had changed at all. Nor had my disease. I had changed. By doing something nice for myself I had lifted my own spirits. I had taken a hand in the course of my treatment, if only by delaying it a week so I could fulfill a dream first. Once again, I had kept breast cancer from taking over my life, and I was glorying in the result. I felt that I was solidly on the right path now. In the three remaining days between my vacation and my mastectomy, I felt better than I had in months. I was facing major surgery and an unknown future, but I didn't feel worried. I was sure I could handle whatever was to come.

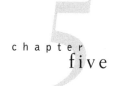

Keep Your Friends Close

*Surround yourself
with people
who make you
feel good.*

Many of us have been brought up to think we are supposed to keep our suffering to ourselves. We learned early that people who talk about their illnesses, who discuss their operations and show off their scars, are tedious, boring, and always to be avoided at parties. But there is a big difference between chattering about your illness to everyone you meet and opening yourself up to the caring support of close friends....

One of the most important decisions a woman with breast cancer has to make is how much of her experience she's going to share. The short-term consequences are obvious. Your decision to include or exclude your friends will determine how much support you get from those closest to you during your health crisis. But there are also long-term consequences that may not be so obvious. How you interact with your friends while you cope with your cancer will influence the shape of your friendships when you return to health.

You may think your doctors and their medical team will provide all the support you need, so you don't have to involve your friends. Doctors certainly have a primary role to play in your recovery, but it is important to see that their ability to help you through the emotional aspects of your breast cancer experience is limited. First of all, the surgeons and oncologists who treat most cancer patients see their disease primarily in physical terms. Even the best doctors—those who understand that an illness like breast cancer is as much a psychological and emotional threat as a physical one—don't have the time or the training to deal with their patients' nonmedical needs. Most doctors are compassionate and many offer advice they hope will help psychologically as well as physically. Unfortunately, in giving psychological advice, they are usually out of their element, and are certainly out of their field of expertise.

It became very clear to me as I went through my cancer treatment that the doctors who understood pretty well what was happening in my body had no idea what was happening in my heart and my mind. Even if I had found a doctor I felt might understand how I was feeling, I don't see how I could have commanded as much of his or her time as it would have taken to connect personally.

Doctors Are Only One Part of Your Team

✿

I had a friend in college who had a theory of horizontal and vertical relationships. The horizontal ones, she said, are those that stretch across long periods of time, that are comfortable and enduring. Vertical relationships, on the other hand, she described as being very intense but lasting for only a short time. She declared both types of relationships to be important and valid, although they are very different. I've thought about her theory a lot over the years, and I think she is right.

I see my relationship with Dr. S. during my breast cancer crisis as a vertical relationship. For a few weeks it was very intense, and extraordinarily intimate. I put my body and my life into his hands. I lay down on a table knowing he was going to cut away my breast, and I wasn't afraid. I trusted him. I believed in him, although I really didn't know him at all. For several weeks afterward I saw him regularly. He removed my bandages, withdrew fluid from my chest, ran his fingers over my body checking the progress of my healing. Then he declared that I was doing fine, and our frequent meetings ceased. Now I see him only three times a year, for about ten minutes. For a few weeks, a few years ago, he was the most important person in my life. If my cancer returns, he may be that important again, but right now he is involved in other lives, not mine.

If I picture my life as a path I am walking, I see Dr. S. as a bridge that carried me safely across a dangerous river, and stayed there to help the next traveler across, as I continued on. On second thought, he was too energetic and powerful in my life to be characterized as a passive bridge. Perhaps I should say he was a lightning bolt that struck when I was lost in darkness and lit my way to safety. In any case, he is gone from my daily life now. Even when he was so powerful an influence, he was with me only for minutes at a time—except in the operating room, and I slept through that encounter.

How much emotional support could he have given me in those few minutes we shared? Not much, I think, despite all good intentions. My realistic sources of support lay in the people I spend significant amounts of time with, in the horizontal relationships that were part of my life before I got sick and continue to be an important part of it now.

Still, in the beginning I felt, as I am sure many other patients do, that doctors must know the best way to deal with the emotions that come with breast cancer; after all, they have dealt with hundreds of women in similar situations before. It wasn't until I began reading books written by doctors that I dropped that illusion. I realized that they are people like the rest of us, shaped and limited by their own experiences, ambitions, and emotions, and by their own struggles to establish meaningful contact with the people close to them.

At one point, after my surgery, I scoured bookstore and library shelves looking for books with insights that would help me absorb and come to terms with the experience I had just been through and the uncertain future I was facing. I was dismayed to find that many books by prominent doctor-authors are poorly written and confusing. Those I read contradicted one another constantly; one contradicted itself from one page to the next. Even worse, some of these leaders in the field of cancer care, who through their books offer guidance to thousands of frightened readers, give out dreadful advice.

One such book suggests that women with breast cancer naturally withdraw from family and friends. "After learning you have cancer, your one and only goal becomes survival," asserts the author, an oncologist and medical school professor who herself had breast cancer. "In an effort to stay alive, you shut yourself off from the rest of the world and its responsibilities. Rarely do you have the will, let alone the desire, to confront the avalanche of emotions that lie behind the supportive smiles of your family and friends." [16] I still get angry when I read those words; I don't think a respected doctor should encourage self-defeating behavior by presenting it as normal.

Once treatment is over, this doctor-author tells her readers, you have to restart your life. "We must look beyond the circle of cancer and reach out to life," she writes, "get back in touch with friends, deal with changes and compromises in our daily lives, and relearn how to interact with members of our own family." I didn't have to go through that. I remained actively involved with the people closest to me throughout my medical crisis, and came out of it with my friendships and family ties stronger and deeper than ever.

Friendship Is Strong Medicine

Fortunately, not all doctors are so far off-base on the importance of close human contact during illness. A number, in fact, have conducted studies in an effort to demonstrate scientifically how emotional support from friends and family helps patients get through a medical crisis. A few of the studies actually turned up the "news," which doesn't surprise me and shouldn't surprise you, that beyond helping a patient's mood, emotional support actually improves a person's chances of survival. Most of the studies dealt with patients who were severely ill or close to death, but it seems to me the same principles would apply as well, if not even more so, to patients who will recover, as most breast cancer patients do.

One study tracked leukemia patients for two years after they underwent bone marrow transplants. At the end of that period, 54 percent of those who said they had strong emotional support from their spouses, family, or friends were still alive, as compared with only 20 percent of those who said they didn't have that kind of support. Another study found that heart patients who had no spouse or close friend were three times as likely to die within five years as those who did have someone close giving them emotional support. [17]

One now-famous study focused on women with breast cancer. All the women included were suffering from advanced metastatic cancer (cancer that had spread beyond the breast) and were expected to die soon. Dr. David Spiegel, a professor of psychiatry at the Stanford University School of Medicine, wanted to see if being part of a support group would help these women to cope with pain and improve their daily lives. He was surprised to find that the women in his support groups not only felt better both physically and psychologically, they lived twice as long as women in the study with the same disease and prognosis who were not in support groups. In interviewing Dr. Spiegel for his 1993 television series "Healing and the Mind," journalist Bill Moyers commented, "When I read about your study, it just seemed so commonsensical that people who get their feelings out in the open, who have the support of loving friends and family, who are able to distract themselves from pain, and who know they are not unique in suffering or alone in dying are going to be happier and more hopeful, and therefore better able to cope with disease." [18]

Moyers is right. It *is* commonsensical, although a lot of people, even doctors, somehow fail to see it. Human contact and emotional support have a great deal to do with anyone's ability to deal with illness. In his conversation with Moyers, Dr. Spiegel expressed hopes that his study would lead to changes in standard practices of medical care. "We have to add to the surgical and medical interventions—which we're doing with increasing skill—a standard component of treatment that involves helping the person who has the disease deal with it and feel supported through it." It is an excellent goal, but I am not sure doctors are ever going to be able to fill the role of emotional support-giver for their patients, or that they should have to. Most of us already have fine emotional support systems in place. All we need to do is call on them.

Friendship Thrives on Sharing

When I think about what friendship can contribute during times of sickness, I can't help thinking also about what sickness can contribute to friendship. We as a culture generally don't see much good in illness. If we grudgingly admit it has anything good to offer, perhaps it is time off from work, a respite from responsibilities. But I cannot avoid the fact that my bout with breast cancer gave me a number of positive things. One of them is that it greatly strengthened my ties to my family and close friends. In that one area at least (and it is not the only one), having breast cancer improved my life.

I know this will sound odd to a lot of people, but I think it's important when you are going through a potentially serious illness like breast cancer to think about how that illness is affecting your friendships and what you can do to make sure its impact is positive. Perhaps you think, *That's crazy. If I am facing a disease that might kill me, I'm going to be thinking about my life, not my friends.* Of course you will be thinking about your life, but what part of your life? Just the part that coincides with your cancer crisis, or all the years beyond? My own cancer crisis lasted from late April 1995, when I discovered a lump in my breast, to late September 1995, when Dr. S. declared me fully healed from my mastectomy. That's five months, not a very big chunk of my life. On the other hand, I have a number of people I have been friends with for more than 20 years. I expect to be close to them for another 30 or 40. Which is more important, an illness that demanded my attention for 5 months or friendships I hope will span 50 years or more?

Fortunately, it is not an either-or proposition. Health and friendship are both extremely important, and it is not only possible, but crucial to tend to both at the same time. The physical and emotional sides of us are intertwined; we are not bodies, we are people. When a disease like breast cancer strikes, it doesn't just intensify our physical needs; it increases our emotional and psychological needs, too. To attend to one and not the others is to throw our lives off balance.

We all know what can happen when people let emotional problems stop them from taking care of themselves physically. Someone is emotionally upset and stops doing positive things such as eating well or sleeping enough, or does harmful things such as smoking or drinking too much. Before long the emotional problem has caused physical damage as well. The same is true when we let physical problems stop us from taking care of ourselves emotionally. Someone upset about having a disease cuts herself off from her friends, or invests her energy in negative emotions like fear and worry. As a result, the disease takes a toll psychologically and emotionally as well as physically.

If you have been diagnosed with breast cancer, you won't have much control over the physical aspects of your illness. Those will be treated by the medical professionals. A woman's main responsibility in that area is to be sure to seek out all the help she needs, to find the best doctors available, and to follow up on tests and treatments to make sure nothing falls through the cracks. All that really doesn't take up very much time, which is good, because although the physical side is pretty well covered, there isn't a whole lot of help available on the psychological/emotional side. That's where you mostly have to do things for yourself. Taking care of the emotional side of your life means keeping your human connections as active and healthy as possible.

Don't Go It Alone

One good source of understanding and support is a breast cancer support group. Strangers who share common problems can quickly become friends. Support groups are especially important for women who are not comfortable talking about cancer with their old friends, or with male friends, and would rather share the experience with women who literally share the experience. If you feel that way and join a cancer support group, I hope you will still allow your healthy friends, male and female, the chance to be with you while you are ill, to distract you from your sickness, and to add new depth to your relationships.

Personally, I am shy among strangers and was not attracted to the idea of a support group. I preferred to share my feelings with people I already knew well. I also did not want my cancer to be the main topic of conversation. Although it was certainly one of the things we talked about, I didn't want my illness to define me, to be the reason for or focus of a relationship.

I began talking to my friends about my possible breast cancer soon after I discovered a lump in my breast. I called a few people specifically to tell them and told others when I happened to see them or when they called about something else. Word got around quickly, and soon friends were calling me to offer sympathy and support. Everyone was concerned, and that made me feel I wasn't facing my crisis alone. I felt like I had a lot of help carrying my worries; when they began to feel overwhelming, I'd call someone and shift a bit to his or her shoulders. Can friends really take worries off your shoulders and carry them for you? I don't know, but each time I shared my fears with a friend I came away feeling that I was carrying less.

I did, however, sense a good deal of uncertainty among my friends. They wanted to help but weren't sure how to go about it. So I told them what I wanted. Time and again I was asked, "Is there anything I can do for you?" Time and again I answered, "I don't need anything in particular. Just don't pull away from me. I need my friends close." Everyone responded. Busy people with very little free time made time to be with me. In the five months of my cancer experience I saw more of my friends than I had in years.

Some of them brought me presents, but their presence was the gift I needed, and treasured. As I look back, I remember Dayna, whose job as a public relations director takes up way too much of her time, sitting on my sofa, chatting casually as if she had all the time in the world. I remember Tim bringing Chinese food to share on his lunch hour on the day I came home from the hospital. I remember, although I wasn't there, Kaila and Willa coming to the house while I was having my mastectomy, bringing flowers for Jay to give to me. The huge bouquet was wonderful, but their real gift was staying with Jay and letting him cook them dinner. Having company and conversation to fill the hours until Dr. S. called to say all had gone well made a huge difference to him.

Of course, all of the conversations Jay and I had with friends during those months included some discussion of breast cancer. I was the first woman in our group of friends to have it, so no one knew very much about it. Once they saw that I was willing to talk openly about cancer, most of our friends had questions. We talked about the physical and the emotional aspects of the disease, comparing the bits and pieces each of us knew, talking about mortality and fear and how having a sick friend affects everybody's outlook. We talked about my surgery, the staples that held my chest together afterward, the pain I had expected that didn't come. The conversations were wide open and very comforting to me. You might think such talks would focus too much of everyone's attention on my illness, but somehow they did the opposite. They separated my cancer from me. They made it a threat that all of us were dealing with, although my particular encounter was more immediate and more intense. I didn't feel isolated in my health crisis because so many people jumped right into it with me, talking about it, sharing their fears, wanting to learn from my experience something that might keep them safer.

Although each of my friends came to these conversations for my sake, nearly every one of them has told me they took something of value away. Friendship is always a two-way street. If you hesitate to call on your friends during your illness, you are not only depriving yourself of their support, you are robbing them of an opportunity to benefit from your experience. I can imagine eyebrows going up. How, exactly, are your friends going to benefit from your being sick? Let me tell you a few of the things that happened. One woman friend in her thirties had never examined her own breasts. She vowed to begin at once. A couple, both of whom work, were shaken by thoughts of their own mortality, which inevitably come up when you see a friend facing a potentially fatal disease. They realized that all of their time was being eaten up by work, chores, and family responsibility. Realizing no one knows how much time he has left, they decided to rearrange their priorities and start making time to spend with friends.

The most surprising, and satisfying, thing to me was that a number of friends told me that after watching me cope with my health crisis they felt they would be better able to handle a crisis of their own should one come up in the future. They said I showed them a different way of being sick, a way they liked. What they meant was that I didn't let my illness consume other parts of my life. I saw my cancer as an intense, temporary experience. I found it frightening, but I also found it interesting and challenging. I talked about it as if it were a fascinating, albeit dangerous journey, which it was. I guess my friends, not knowing much about breast cancer, expected to find me after my mastectomy in pain, in bed, and in need of cheering up. Instead I was upbeat and energetic, planning outings and urging them to come along. Who says having a serious disease means you have to stop enjoying life? You can still have fun and be fun.

Tim's Approach

In truth, I myself wondered sometimes where I got the idea that being sick doesn't mean you have to act sick. It struck me one day that my attitude toward sickness stems from a lesson I learned many years ago from my friend Tim, a rather unconventional thinker and one of the wisest people I have ever known.

Tim is a musician. Back in the '70s he always seemed to be going to one concert or another. Sometimes I went with him. On one occasion he, his girlfriend Julie, and I bought tickets to hear Talking Heads, but when the day of the concert arrived I was suffering from an abscessed tooth. My dentist had been unable to tell which tooth was abscessed, so he had sent me home to wait until the pain "localized." It localized all right, and increased to an unbearable agony. I had an appointment to have it taken care of the next morning. In the meantime, the only thing that lessened the pain was holding ice on the spot. I had been lying on my sofa since late afternoon popping shards of ice into my mouth. I called Tim to tell him I wouldn't be able to go to the concert.

His response shocked me. "You're going to be in pain wherever you are," he said, "so why not come to the concert and have a good time? I never would have looked at the situation that way, but as soon as he said it, I knew he was right. I protested that I didn't want to make him and Julie uncomfortable. "It's not going to affect us," he said. I knew Tim well enough to believe him. My pain was mine, not his. There was nothing he could do about it, so he wouldn't let it stop him from having fun.

I went to the concert, armed with an insulated picnic bag full of ice, which I steadily fed into my mouth. During intermission Tim and Julie went to the lobby for drinks; they brought back paper cups of ice to replenish my supply. The band was terrific and we all had a great time. I spent the rest of the night alone, in pain, and miserable. Each time I put a piece of ice in my mouth the pain would subside and I would fall asleep. Within seconds the ice would melt and the pain would return and wake me up. I don't think I slept more than two minutes all night long. When I look back on that night, I remember how devastating the pain felt as I lay alone on the sofa, and how insignificant it seemed as I sat with Tim and Julie listening to Talking Heads. That night my attitude toward pain and illness changed forever.

Go Fly a Kite

I had my mastectomy late on a Wednesday afternoon and came home from the hospital the following morning. Two long surgical tubes stuck out of my chest, draining fluid into a pair of plastic vacuum bottles. With all this apparatus attached to me it was hard to find a comfortable position for my body, especially in bed at night. Pinning the bottles to my clothes, as a nurse had suggested, made me feel like a small child was constantly tugging at me, wanting something. It wasn't painful, just constantly annoying, and I knew it wasn't going to go away for at least a week.

Suddenly I remembered the purple fanny pack I'd gotten the previous Christmas and had stuffed in a drawer. I dug around and found it buried under some scarves and gloves. The bottles fit in perfectly. I could even coil the extra length of tubing on top. The pack made the bottles seem weightless and kept them out of my way. Now I could sit; I could lie down; I felt free.

That Saturday was the annual Berkeley Kite Festival in the park down by the marina. A kite festival may sound pretty low-key, but it's actually a dazzling event. Colorful, high-tech kites, singly and in groups, perform choreographed dances to music high above the heads of the audience, who sprawl on the grass snacking, cheering, and generally being proud of themselves for having discovered this delightfully wacky entertainment. Jay and I invited our friends Mike and Kaila to come with us.

"Are you sure?" they asked. "So soon after surgery? "

I told them we were going, whether they came or not. They came. I tucked my plastic bottles into my fanny pack and off we went. Before long we all were so caught up in the show we forgot about my surgery.

A friend I hadn't seen in a while spotted us lounging on the grass and came over to say hi. She asked what was new, so I told her about my mastectomy. She looked skeptical. I unzipped my fanny pack and showed her my bottles.

"What are you doing here?" she gasped.

"Where should I be?" I replied. "At home, being miserable?"

Several months later that friend's husband underwent surgery for a brain tumor. A few months after his ordeal our families went hiking together at Yosemite. As we made our way back down the trail, Jack and I lagged behind the others, talking about our illnesses. I had to remind him about my cancer experience. Although we had talked several times since my surgery, the subject hadn't come up and he had totally forgotten that I too had had cancer. We talked about the support we had both gotten from family and friends, and about how much more alive we felt after confronting the possibility of our death. It was a sparkling day and we found it hard to keep our minds on illness in such a spectacularly beautiful place. Our conversation soon turned to the mountains and then to how fast our children were growing, his red-haired son and my red-haired daughter, romping not far ahead of us on the trail. Cancer faded from our minds. It was just something that had happened to us both that didn't seem very important to either of us any more.

Do as Much as Feels Right to You

Every woman dealing with breast cancer has to find her own level of comfortable activity. If you come out of surgery and are tired and in pain, you are probably not going to want to stuff your surgical bottles in a fanny pack and take off for your local equivalent of a kite festival. On the other hand, perhaps you should. I can't believe there is any pain more excruciating than an abscessed tooth, and I sure felt better at the height of my agony being with friends at a concert. As my friend Tim had predicted, the pain wasn't any better, but my life was better.

I have heard it said that with a disease like cancer you are always alone. You are the one facing it, not your family or friends. I totally disagree. You are alone only to the extent to which you choose to face your crisis alone. Some women keep their feelings to themselves, thinking they are protecting those they love. You cannot protect the people close to you from the effects of your illness. The fact that you are ill affects them. If you keep them at a distance during your ordeal, you will be depriving them of an opportunity to deal with their own emotions, to learn from your experience, and to strengthen the bonds between you.

Times of crisis offer great opportunities for building deeper relationships. We are all so busy in our everyday lives, most of us don't spend too much time cultivating intimacy. Our interactions with friends tend to stay on the surface, providing pleasant moments but doing little to reinforce deep connections. I love to go out for a drink or a movie with a friend or to chat on the phone or share a nice dinner, but I am often aware that we don't have the time or the right setting to dig deep into each other's lives.

All that changes when one of you is plunged into a crisis. Suddenly emotions are raw and close to the surface. Confronted with strong emotions, a friend has two choices—to pull away or to connect. Real friends connect. I am not referring to your friend, I am referring to you. You are the friend who must reach out, because in most cases your friends will be reluctant to push too hard. They will wait for a signal from you to tell them if you want intimacy or you want to go it alone. Choose intimacy. The energy that is ignited inside both people when that connection is made is powerful, positive, and unforgettable; the bonds of friendship that are forged remain strong long after cancer is forgotten.

Welcome Your Family's Support

*Don't shut out
your family,
especially children.*

Sometimes, in our efforts to protect the ones we love, we hurt them instead. When I was 6 years old, my 8-year-old brother, my only sibling, died of bone cancer. His illness was relatively brief. It started with a pain in his arm. The doctors diagnosed cancer and amputated the arm at the shoulder. But the cancer had already spread to his lungs. Within six months he was dead....

During Buddy's last days in the hospital, I was not allowed to see him. As soon as he died, I was sent to stay with family friends in another state. I was not allowed to attend his funeral or to be at home during the week of mourning that followed.

I know that my parents were trying to protect me. I also know, after talking about it with my mother many years later, that she was so overwhelmed with her own emotions that she never stopped to think that I had emotional needs too. Young, frightened, and bewildered, I had to deal with my feelings alone. I couldn't handle them, so I sealed them, and my memories of them, away somewhere beyond reach. To this day, I can remember nothing of my brother and almost nothing at all of the first six years of my life.

I long ago forgave my parents for excluding me from the family during that crisis, but I still feel the pain when I think about it. If you think you will save your children pain by shielding them from your illness, you are fooling yourself, and shortchanging them.

Your Kids Are Tuned In

I think in general parents tend to underestimate their children—not only their needs, but also their level of awareness. Kids, even very young ones, are perceptive. They notice and understand a lot more than adults give them credit for. If there is a shift in the atmosphere in the house, if there is unusual tension in the air, they sense it no matter how hard you try to hide it. They may not say anything, but they know something is not right and they worry about it. Their sense of security is shaken. If they are not let in on the "secret," the truth of what is going on, they try to figure it out for themselves, using their limited experience of the adult world and their very vivid imaginations. Often they imagine something far worse than what is actually happening, and they become frightened. Because kids are naturally self-centered, they may also decide that whatever is wrong must somehow be their fault.

When it comes to which subjects are open for discussion within the family and which ones are not, kids usually take their cue from their parents. They wait for an adult to begin the conversation. If it is obvious to them that their parents don't want to talk about something, they are not likely to bring it up either. So it is up to you, the adult, to decide how much information you want your kids to have and when you want to begin sharing your experience with them. The important thing is that you think about them and their emotional needs from the start. What you decide to say is probably going to be less important than the fact that you are paying attention to their feelings and trying to respond to them. In the end, each parent knows her own kids and her personal capacities for communication better than anyone else. Helping your kids through your health crisis is a very personal and individual challenge.

Talking with Rebecca

✿

My daughter, Rebecca, was 8 years old when I discovered the lumps in my breast. I began thinking immediately about how much to tell her and when. On one hand, I didn't want to worry her if it was going to turn out that I was all right. On the other, if something was seriously wrong with me, I was determined not to exclude her and leave her to deal with her emotions alone.

I decided initially to hold off until I knew there was actually something wrong with me. For the first month after I found my lumps, my tests were inconclusive and my doctors optimistic. Then, in early June, a needle aspiration, my third test, turned up "atypical" cells and I was told a surgical biopsy would be necessary. I felt then that the time had come to talk to Rebecca.

I sat down with her and said—very simply, I thought—"There is something I need to tell you." I felt her antennae shoot up, searching for emotional clues to what was going on and how she should react. I moved ahead cautiously, making sure my voice stayed calm, as if I were explaining plans for a trip we were going to take together. I said there were two lumps in my breast and that the doctors were going to take them out. I pulled up my shirt and showed her where the lumps were. I encouraged her to feel them. I didn't mention cancer during that first conversation. Since Dr. R. had said that whether the lumps were malignant or not, after the biopsy they'd be gone, I honestly thought that simple operation would be the end of it, for both of us.

I tried to think of what might worry Rebecca and to concentrate on those things. I told her I would not be staying in the hospital overnight and that I did not expect to be sick afterwards. I said I would probably be tired, though, so she might need to help out more than usual. She seemed glad to have an easy way to respond. She said she would help Daddy take care of everything when I came home so I could rest. I thanked her and said that would be terrific. As she left the room I felt good. I had told her enough to make her feel she was part of what was happening and had given her a role to play, all, it seemed, without alarming her.

I did come home from the biopsy feeling a little tired, but otherwise was fine. When I removed the bandage a few days later I was shocked to see that almost a third of my breast was bright purple. It was a truly amazing bruise, and my exclamations brought both Jay and Rebecca into the bathroom to take a look. We all declared it the biggest, most garishly colorful bruise we had ever seen. It occurred to me that the bruise provided a way for Rebecca and me to share my experience. It became sort of a mother-daughter science project. We checked it out together each day to see how it was fading and what colors came through as it healed. I invited Rebecca to touch my breast, but for the first few days she held back. Then one day she said she wanted to touch it. She ran her fingers ever so gently over the bruise and the stitches in the middle of it. It was a special moment that made me feel very close to my daughter.

A week after the biopsy I got the news that my lumps were malignant and I was facing a mastectomy. Rebecca and I sat down to talk again. I tried to sound matter-of-fact as I told her things had changed. The doctors had found out there was still something bad in my breast and the whole breast would have to be removed. I said, for the first time, that the lumps were cancer. She sucked in her breath and her eyes grew wide in panic. She obviously had heard enough about cancer somewhere to be frightened by it.

I talked as calmly as I could, watching her intently as she began to relax. I explained that I was having the operation to stop the cancer before it spread, so that I could be healthy and strong again. I told her I wasn't worried about losing my breast and that she shouldn't worry either. I told her I'd be the same old mom afterwards, except I'd have only one breast. I pointed out jokingly that she was through with my breasts anyway. She said she still liked them. I assured her that one would be enough for cuddling purposes, and explained that I didn't have much choice. My health was more important than the breast. She agreed, we hugged, and on we went.

This new stage of my cancer experience caused disruptions in our family's normal schedule, including Rebecca's. It was summer and she was going to day camp, which ended at 3 in the afternoon. Jay started coming with me to medical appointments, which always seemed to fall late in the afternoon, so we had to ask friends to look after Rebecca. If she hadn't known what was going on, I would have had to come up with some plausible explanation. As it was, I could say, "Daddy and I have to see a surgeon to get a second opinion; you are going to stay with Alison and Julian until we get back." That was all she needed to know, and as long as we didn't seem upset, she wasn't either.

We were lucky that Rebecca was invited to an overnight party the day of my mastectomy, so she was off with friends having fun during what was, for me, the tensest time of the entire ordeal. I'm not sure what we would have done otherwise. I guess she would have been home with Jay, and he would have tried to make it as normal an afternoon and evening as possible, while waiting nervously for word from the hospital. The party was a much better alternative, and I think I would advise families to send their kids off with friends if possible during the actual time of surgery and the inevitable tension of waiting to hear whether it has gone well.

Kids Love Being Treated Like Friends

I came home from the hospital the next morning, and Rebecca came home from her party shortly thereafter. I don't think she felt that I had even been away. I was home, as usual, when she returned; she was the one who had been away. Since I was not in pain, I didn't need to put up a brave front for her benefit. Once again we shared the strange physical aftermath of surgery. I showed her all my medical apparatus—the tubes and bottles and bandages—and we talked about how I was going to cope with them.

Over the next few weeks she became very familiar with my daily routines of removing dressings, draining fluid that accumulated in my chest after the tubes were gone, and taping on new dressings. I left the bathroom door open so that she could wander in and watch if she wanted. I didn't want her to feel that something terrible was going on that I was hiding from her. When there were things that were awkward for me to do alone, like taping a dressing, she helped, cautiously at first, then with growing pride in her ability to assist me. She watched with amusement and offered advice when Jay got into the act, washing my hair for me in the sink during the time when I wasn't allowed to shower or take a bath.

In the weeks after surgery I made many trips to the hospital to have fluid drained from my chest. In order for it to heal completely, the thin outer flap of skin and tissue that had once covered my breast had to adhere to the muscles of the chest wall. That couldn't happen so long as fluid kept filling the space in between. Dr. S. drew the fluid out with a syringe every two or three days, but it kept coming back. He didn't want to let it build up over the weekends, so he asked the resident surgeon at the hospital to do the honors on Saturday or Sunday. Rebecca came with me to those strange weekend meetings in the deserted surgery department. I wanted her to see how ordinary and boring the process was, to see that there was nothing mysterious or frightening about it. I am sure she would have imagined something much worse if she hadn't gotten to see it. In all honesty, I also appreciated her company. It's not a lot of fun hanging around an empty hospital lobby on a Sunday morning wondering if a busy young surgeon is going to remember your rendezvous.

All Dr. S.'s efforts to get my chest to heal were in vain, and eventually he inserted a new surgical tube, which drained fluid into a dressing constantly for a week and did the trick. When I ran out of official surgical dressings, I bought diapers, which I cut in half and secured over the tube. Rebecca, my steadfast assistant, thought that a clever solution. Eventually we gave the leftover diapers to the baby sister of one of her soccer teammates.

Rebecca and I don't talk much about my operation any more. She is used to seeing my lopsided torso and thinks nothing of it. One day she and I looked at a poster of a woman who had a flower stem tattoo obscuring her mastectomy scar. I had considered a tattoo myself at one point. I asked Rebecca what she thought.

"You don't need it," she said. "You look fine the way you are." I agreed.

The only other time my one-breastedness comes up is when we are cuddling on the sofa, reading or watching TV. If she's on my left, she sometimes asks to switch places. "I'm on your hard side," she says. "Your soft side is more comfortable to lean on." We switch.

My prognosis was good following the mastectomy, so I have not talked to Rebecca about the dire consequences of advanced breast cancer. I hope I won't have to. But if my cancer recurs someday, she will be one of the first to know, and we will handle whatever happens together. I know that one day I will also have to talk to her about heredity and what my illness may imply about her future. I would like to wait until she is a teenager, but she'll probably read this first, and I'll have to talk about it sooner.

My cancer and her risk are family matters, burdens we share. We cannot change our genes, so we will have to face whatever comes. I feel that we have laid the groundwork. In facing my illness together, we reduced the scary breast cancer monster to a manageable inconvenience, and we proved our commitment to taking care of each other. All parents get to take care of sick kids. Sometimes kids get to help sick parents. It's not the kind of experience you look for, but neither should you avoid it when it happens.

When Rebecca was very young I promised her that I would never lie to her. I have repeated that promise several times as she has grown older. I want her to know she can trust me, and that I will always try to help her through whatever she has to face. I think hiding my illness from her would have been lying to her, and I think it would have been selling her short. She may have been only 8 years old when my cancer struck, but she had a lot of love and caring to offer. I think it was important for both of us that I accepted it and honestly appreciated it.

Breaking Through to Your Partner

Dealing with a child's response to a serious illness is, in many ways, easier than dealing with an adult's. Most children haven't yet learned to hide their emotions; many adults, especially men, are experts at it. When a woman comes home with the news that she has breast cancer, what goes through her partner's mind? The first reaction after the initial shock has to be a fear of losing her. The word *cancer* triggers images of death in most of our minds.

The day I returned from my postbiopsy consultation with the news that I had cancer, I burst into the house, into tears, and into Jay's arms, seemingly all at once. I'm sure he was as stunned by the news as I was, and as frightened, but he didn't show his fear. I suspect it's easier for two women to share their honest feelings in such an emotionally charged situation, but men in our society have been taught that they have a role to play. Jay was the husband, the strong one, the solid pillar there for me to cling to as I sobbed. He held me gently and let me cry, while he must have felt his world crashing down along with mine.

By the time I stopped crying and was able to look at him, he was calm and rational. His emotions, whatever they were, had already been hidden away, perhaps because he felt he had to be strong for me, perhaps because he didn't want to face them. We sat down at the kitchen table to talk medical facts and to plan our next step.

During the next few days, I broke down and cried many times, but Jay was absolutely stoic. He was always available to listen, to accompany me to medical appointments, and to help me plan for my upcoming surgery, but he showed no strong feelings about what was going on. His mind was accessible; his emotions were not. I began to feel, despite his unfailing attentiveness, that he had deserted me. I would be sitting at my desk trying to fend off the waves of fear, self-doubt, and distress about our uncertain future, while he was sitting at his desk, calmly engrossed in writing his newspaper column. Finally I could stand it no longer. I tramped determinedly down the stairs to his office and said I had to know how he was feeling about my having cancer. He answered casually that he didn't think about it very much. "It doesn't really affect my life like it does yours," he said. I exploded.

All my frustrations with his silence came rushing out.

"It does affect your life," I told him. I think I was shouting. "What happens to me affects you. If I die and you become a single parent, it's going to affect you tremendously. If I get very sick, that's going to affect you. My cancer is your problem as well as mine."

He gave me a look I'd seen before and have seen many times since. It was a look that said, "I can see I'm not going to be able to avoid this one." He set his work aside and we went into the kitchen to talk it out.

There are many difficult areas in marriage. I think communication is the most difficult of all. It has been said many times that men and women do not communicate in the same language, and I think that is true. Women, as a rule, talk about their problems to share them; they look for understanding and emotional support. Most men are far more pragmatic and solution-oriented. They think of problems as something to solve, not something to share. If there is no solution, then what's the point of talking about the problem?

Besides being a typical male in this area, Jay also comes from a family that avoids talking about emotionally charged subjects whenever possible. Early in our relationship, when we were just roommates and not yet romantically involved, I became frustrated with the way he would seek my advice for his emotional (girlfriend) problems, but disappear when I had a problem I wanted to talk about. I attributed such behavior to self-centeredness and an insensitivity to other people's emotions, and told him so. He stunned me by agreeing that I was right and promising to change.

I remember looking at him in amazement and thinking, wow, there's a lot more to this guy than I thought. Since then he has worked hard at learning to recognize and respond to other people's emotions, especially mine, and he has grown into a deep, warm, loving, and loveable man. Still, for all his considerable progress, he wasn't prepared for the emotional demands of breast cancer. Who ever is? Confronted with my health crisis, he had backslid into "not seeing" emotions he didn't know how to handle, both mine and his, telling himself there was nothing he could do about the situation, so what was the point of worrying about it?

The point, I told him in no uncertain terms, was that I needed him with me. I needed all of him, not just his body to hug and his mind to help me plan. I needed more of him than I had ever needed before. I needed his support and his concern and his compassion and his fears and his bewilderment. I wasn't looking for answers, I was looking for a partner. For better or for worse, till death do us part. Silence was not acceptable. Denying that my cancer was his problem too was not acceptable. I couldn't go on flinging my emotions at his calm facade and not go crazy. I wanted to feel his emotions coming back at me, even if they were charged with the frustration, confusion, and terror that were making him hide from them. I wanted, needed, to feel that he was there, every bit of him, good and bad, weak and strong, rational and angry, emotionally alive.

I got through to him. I could see him looking deep into himself as he began talking haltingly about his fear of losing me and about feeling overwhelmed by the possibility of having to bring Rebecca up by himself. We talked for a good half hour and didn't solve a single problem. What we did accomplish was to begin taking down the wall that had been growing between us and separating us. It was only the first of many honest, open conversations about breast cancer and our future. It was in some ways the hardest, and in many ways the most satisfying. Going into it I didn't know if I could break through to him, and I dreaded the isolation ahead of me if I failed. Coming out, I was jubilant. I knew I had my husband back. Cancer might still destroy our lives, but it wasn't going to destroy our relationship. Whatever lay ahead, I knew we were in it together.

Emotional Sensitivity Is a Side Effect of Cancer

I cannot overemphasize how important it was to me that Jay stopped shutting me out of his feelings about my illness. I know it was good for him, too, to face his own fears and feelings of helplessness. From a simple health standpoint, it is bad to bury strong feelings. When my brother got cancer and then died, my father could not express his anguish. He held his feelings inside, where they sent his blood pressure sky high. Jay's father has had serious heart trouble, and I always worry that Jay may follow suit. No woman facing cancer needs to add to her worries a concern that her condition may cause her partner's health to suffer. More important even than health, however, is that very basic, mysterious, vulnerable connection that holds a couple together—the "relationship."

Breast cancer has been known to destroy marriages. Usually husbands will stick around until the crisis has passed. When things calm down again, some of them leave. A few tell their wives they no longer find them attractive after mastectomy, or even that they find their bodies offensive. But those are the brutes, the shallow, arrogant, immature men any woman is better off without. The sad cases are the relationships that are worth having but that crumble under the physical, emotional, and psychological pressures of serious illness.

One of the side effects of cancer that no doctor warned me about is that the stress makes you emotionally supersensitive to the people around you. Silences, as I discovered, are suddenly deafening. Coolness in your partner's manner chills you to the bone. His refusal to talk feels like a slap in the face. In some ways a health crisis like breast cancer is like a bright light trained on your relationship. If there are flaws, they show up. The weak spots you never noticed suddenly become painfully obvious. Small offenses look bigger; innocent oversights appear deliberate. Looking at your husband in such harsh light, you may see things you do not like, as he may see things he does not like in you.

Some marriages simply cannot survive the scrutiny. For most, I believe, the situation, as negative as it may seem, can turn out to be an opportunity to reaffirm your commitment to each other and to shore up any weak spots you find in the relationship.

Throughout my illness my marriage felt more important to me than my health crisis. I had faith that somehow I would survive the cancer. My biggest worry was not that I would die, but that I might lose the closeness Jay and I had worked so hard to build. If that happened, I feared I might lose him. I know a lot of women simply accept their husbands' reluctance to talk openly about their emotions. I am not one to accept that kind of behavior. I knew it was hard for Jay to face his feelings, but life is hard, and good relationships are both difficult to come by and well worth fighting for. I cannot tell other women what to do, but I can say that I am glad I went after the emotional support I needed. Our marriage is even stronger now than it was before my illness.

All Kinds of Families

I think I need to say something here about my definition of family, which may be, probably is, different from yours. All the time I was growing up, my parents, and therefore I, had very limited interactions with aunts, uncles, cousins, and other relatives. For me, "family" always meant immediate family. At the time of my brother's illness, my family included just him, me, and our parents. When my own cancer occurred many years later, I had a much closer relationship with my husband's family than I had ever had with my own, but we didn't have daily, or even weekly contact, so to me "family" still meant immediate family—this time me, my husband, and my daughter. It is, happily, a close and loving family, but very small.

Your definition of family, and your actual household, may include many more people than mine. If so, you're even better off. If you see your parents, grandparents, in-laws, grandchildren, cousins, aunts, and uncles frequently, or even daily, you will be able to spread any extra work among them, and bask in the added attention. I've always envied big, close families. If you have one, count yourself lucky, and take full advantage of all the warmth and support it offers.

If you live alone, or with a partner, as many women do, your family is different from mine in yet another way. It doesn't matter who you include in your concept of family. The people you live with and any others who are part of your inner family circle are the most important in helping you to get through your crisis.

Regardless of the support you get from doctors and friends, it is your family that is with you day in and day out, when you're feeling energetic and when you're exhausted, when you're optimistic and when you're not sure you can face another day. The members of your family cannot escape the reality of your illness. They are there, in the same room or the next room; their lives cannot help but be affected. It is important to see that while you need extra attention because of your illness, so do they.

Care for Your Family
While They Care for You

While your family members are pitching in to take care of you physically, be sure you are doing your part to take care of them, as well as yourself, emotionally and psychologically. Sickness can be as much of a threat to family relationships as it is to the body of the person struck by disease. For one thing, illness provides lots of opportunities for guilt. You feel guilty because your sickness is disrupting the lives of those closest to you. They feel guilty because they want to continue their own activities but feel obligated to give more of their time and attention to you.

Guilt is not unlike cancer. It starts small, with just a word or even a look. Once it takes root, its poison spreads. Like most Jewish women, I know a lot about guilt. When I was a child it was spoon-fed to me with my breakfast cereal, and even now that I am in my 50s, it is a major presence in most of my conversations with my mother. I hate guilt. I refuse to use it or to let it enter any relationships over which I have control. It is important to recognize guilt's destructive power and to be on the lookout for it.

Your illness is not your fault. It is not your family's fault either. It is one of those things that happen, and it has happened to you and your family. The fact that you are sick will, of course, put some pressure on everyone in your family, but the physical changes that may be unavoidable need not cause emotional strain. You may need your husband, or son or daughter, to drive you to doctor's appointments or pick up some of your household chores temporarily. You don't need them to stop living their own lives, or to put your needs constantly above their own. Tell them so. Tell them you appreciate the extra attention they are giving you and that you will certainly do the same for them when they go through tough times in their lives. Love and communication keep family relationships healthy; guilt and sacrifice, especially reluctant sacrifice, tear them apart.

When you are ill it is sometimes hard to focus on anything else. Cancer patients have been known to let their disease become the only subject of their conversations. Be sure to ask other family members about what is going on in their lives while they are away from the house or away from you. Your husband's and children's activities will probably be a lot more fun to talk about anyway, and they will like getting the attention. Don't let your sickness become a black hole that sucks conversation into it and drains joy and laughter from the family. Even on your worst days, you'll feel better talking about the enjoyable things others are doing.

Keep in mind that your cancer crisis will probably pass; your family life will continue on. It is easier to keep family relationships healthy than to damage or neglect them during your illness and try to patch them up afterwards. When you are well again, you and your family will still feel good about each other—perhaps even better than before—and will be able to congratulate yourselves on how well you weathered the storm.

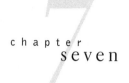
Stoke Your Appetite for Life

Think about all you have to live for.

It's become so common, most people hardly even notice that the vocabulary we use in talking about disease is a vocabulary of war. Sick people are victims fighting off illnesses that threaten to destroy them. Doctors prescribe treatments to attack and kill viruses, bacteria, and invasive cancer cells. When a cancer patient recovers her good health, she is said to have won the battle of (and for) her life. She is a survivor....

They are only words, you may say, but the vocabulary we use has tremendous influence on the way we think. This particular vocabulary encourages us to see our bodies as battlefields, relentlessly stalked, as are all battlefields, by the threat of death. It focuses too much of our attention on images of a desperate fight against a powerful enemy and not enough on our positive motivations for getting well, chief among them our love of life.

I have never been comfortable with either the reality or the metaphors of war, or with any kind of violence for that matter. When I first realized that cancer was threatening my life, I was determined not to dwell on thoughts of death or think of my body as waging war against an internal enemy. I thought any negative feelings—especially fear and anger—would work against me, so I tried to banish them from my mind. Despite all my efforts, they kept sneaking back and overwhelming me. It took some time for me to realize that those negative emotions were as much a part of my natural response to my sickness as the positive, optimistic ones I preferred. My dark feelings were contributing in their own way to my efforts to survive and to heal.

Fear of Death
Feeds the Will To Live

I tried at first to suppress my fear, speaking of it only to my husband, and only when I could not hold it back anymore. I was afraid that if I gave in to it, I would lose control and be reduced to that dreadful stereotype, a helpless female crying uncontrollably and unable to act in her own behalf. The fear kept returning, of course, and eventually I gave up trying to deny it or fight it off. Funny how a change of attitude can change your perspective. Once I accepted my fear, I began to see it in an entirely different way. It occurred to me that fear doesn't have to be the negative, debilitating emotion we assume it is. In many ways it is a positive, natural reaction to danger, designed to keep us on our toes and keep us safe.

Instinctive fear is one of nature's great gifts. When we sense that we are in immediate physical danger, it can trigger a shot of adrenaline that provides the extra measure of strength or speed we need to save ourselves and/or others. Obviously, a sudden burst of strength or speed will not save anyone from cancer, but fear contributes to our self-preservation in other ways as well.

I remember being overcome by fear only once before my bout with cancer. Jay and I were on vacation in Italy. We stood at the mouth of a narrow tunnel on a country road at twilight. He said we had to walk through it to get to a restaurant on the other side. Cars were racing by in both directions, and it seemed to me that if a car came through while we were inside, there wouldn't be enough room to press our bodies against the tunnel wall and avoid being hit. I refused to enter. No amount of arguing could change my mind, because it wasn't my mind that was in charge. It was my instinct. Luckily, a car came along going in our direction and the driver offered us a ride. The problem was solved and I quickly regained my good spirits, but I have never forgotten that tunnel or the fear that kept me out of it.

When you are faced with a serious illness, the fear that grips you is also generated by your instinct to survive. The fear itself can be terrifying, but if you accept it as a positive response to a dangerous situation, it can work in your favor, helping to focus your energies in a wondrous phenomenon called "the will to live." I'm not going to pretend I know just what the will to live is. Nobody seems to know what it is, where it comes from, why some people have more of it than others, or how it affects the way our bodies function. But many people, including doctors, have come to recognize its importance, because they have seen people who have it—ordinary people in every other way—bounce back from serious illnesses that should, according to medical expectations, have been the end of them.

Whether your cancer is diagnosed at an early, curable stage or is already advanced, you want to give yourself every possible chance of recovery, which means you'll need all of your body's natural fighting and healing energies working at capacity. What appears to get them going and keep them going is the will to live, so it is very important that you find yours, and keep it stoked.

Positive *and* Negative Emotions Play a Role

How do you jump-start your will to live and make sure it's working in your favor? I believe you do it by opening yourself up to both positive *and* negative feelings and letting them stir up your appetite for life.

In the days following my cancer diagnosis I felt constantly battered by waves of emotion—intense love and fear and a whole range of only slightly less powerful feelings, including anger, sadness, courage, and desperation. I kept telling myself to "get a grip" and forced myself to be unemotional in those situations where I thought calm was required. I was proud of myself for sitting patiently in hospital waiting rooms. I patted myself on the back for being able to talk sensibly with doctors and ask pertinent questions. I stunned myself with my ability to walk calmly down long hospital corridors moments before my mastectomy, while an anesthesiologist I had met only moments before explained in a soft voice how she was going to put me out. I did all of these things, perfectly under control, because I believed it was required.

When I was at home and at work, it was a different story. As I sat at my desk, my emotions clearly had the upper hand. My daughter's face would flash before me and I would be ripped by longing to be with her forever. Or I would see myself lying in a hospital bed, near death, and my heart would feel crushed by sadness. My hands would go limp on the keyboard and I would close my eyes, waiting for the storm to pass. I probably would have stopped those emotions if I had known how. Yet even while I was hating them, on some level I knew they were appropriate. I also had other reasons for wanting to endure the onslaught.

In the past, I'd been much too successful in suppressing my emotions. At the tender age of six, unable to cope with my brother's death, I had learned to bury my feelings. For years I continued that pattern, gradually walling myself into a relentlessly grey world where strong emotions were neither felt nor expressed. As an adult, living in a more nurturing environment than the one I grew up in, I began to feel that an important part of me was missing, and I began a long, hard struggle to find and release my emotions, especially the negative ones. By the time I was stricken with cancer I had made considerable progress and was determined not to backslide, despite the immense force of the feelings that assaulted me. I wanted to feel them. At the time I was thinking more about my mental health than my physical health, but in retrospect I am convinced that all the time those powerful, upsetting, wrenching emotions were battering me, they were also feeding my determination to beat my cancer.

If you are facing cancer, or any other serious illness, don't be surprised by the fact that you feel angry, scared, sad, and desperate. Those are appropriate emotions. They are not negative, outside forces attacking you; they spring from efforts of your own mind and body to stimulate your fighting spirit.

Some people will tell you that it is silly and a waste of energy to get angry at your disease or the capriciousness of fate. Don't listen. Get angry. Doctors and medical researchers have found that people who get angry at their illness are more likely to successfully fight it off than people who resign themselves to it. [19]

When well-meaning friends and relatives tell you not to allow yourself to think about the possibility of dying, ignore their advice. When the fear of death hits you, stop what you're doing and think about the terrible and terrifying truth that this disease might indeed kill you. Think about all the people and things you will lose if you die. Let yourself fill up with the aching, the longing for everything you love, and then refuse to die.

What Do You Live For?

When I thought about dying, my first thoughts were always of my husband and daughter. I thought of how much I loved them both, and how much they needed me to be around. Rebecca was nearing her ninth birthday, no longer a little girl but still far from ready to face the world without a mother's help. I couldn't bear the thought of her growing up without me. There were so many things I needed to tell her. I thought about her as a teenager, trying to cope with her own changing emotions and the fast-paced world outside, and I ached to be there for her.

I felt just as strongly about my husband. Jay is the man I thought would never enter my life. He came late, when I was already 37 years old. We built our love slowly and carefully, and I was 41 when we finally married. After seemingly endless years of loneliness and struggle, I was with a man who understood me, who laughed with me and occasionally fought with me, made me feel attractive, and let me know every day that I was unconditionally loved. The 10 years of our marriage had zoomed by; I wanted at least 20 or 30 more.

Each time I got together with friends during those months, I realized how much they, too, meant to me, and how I would hate to lose them. I had made a concerted effort for more than 20 years to build a warm and nurturing circle around me. My friends are fascinating people whose lives are always changing, and I wanted to see what was coming next for them. I wanted to hear the music Tim was writing and see the paintings Dan was working on in his new little studio. I wanted to see if Dayna and Scott were really going to have kids, and what kind of kids they would be. I wanted to stand on Susan and Matt's newly built deck on the Fourth of July and watch the fireworks over San Francisco Bay, not just the next year, but year after year. I simply wasn't ready to die.

As I thought about all the wonderful people in my life, I realized that the person I was least happy with was myself. I had accomplished some good things, but I wasn't the person I wanted to be. I think each of us has an image of who we are, deep down inside. For many of us, the life we end up living is not the life of that deep-down person. Deep inside I always saw myself as a writer, someone who tries to understand and explore what's true and important in life. I was, in fact, a writer of sorts. I had co-authored two cookbooks. I could bang out a dynamite press release. I had written countless pamphlets and newsletters, ads and catalog blurbs, and even a number of magazine articles, but I was not writing about the things that were most important to me, or even subjects I particularly cared about. I had slipped into writing simply to be paid.

To give myself some credit, about six years before my cancer diagnosis I had stopped working as a writer-for-hire to concentrate on book editing. Jay and I started our own small cookbook publishing company. It gave us independence and felt to me like a major step in regaining control over my life. But when I looked at my situation from the new perspective my cancer gave me, I saw how far I still was from realizing my dreams. Instead of being a copywriter, I was a publisher and an editor—an independent publisher, and a very good editor—but still not what I wanted to be.

I was shaken by the thought that I might die without ever becoming the person I could have, should have, been. I was angry with myself for having gotten sidetracked. The more I thought about it, the more determined I became to beat my damn cancer and go out and take a real shot, once and for all, at being a writer. And so, much to my surprise, at the same time I was worrying about dying, I became excited about the future.

People who have never gone through a life-threatening illness find it hard to believe that it can be a positive experience. And yet, for many cancer patients, including myself, it has been just that. I dreaded the changes breast cancer would make in my life, but it turned out that the most significant changes it brought are good ones for which I am grateful. It sounds like a contradiction—the terrible disease that opens the door to a wonderful future—but life is full of contradictions, and many dark clouds have silver linings. The sudden, rigorous self-examination which I and many other cancer patients have experienced is a positive and very powerful side effect of the disease.

In her book *Revolution from Within*, Gloria Steinem reveals that her bout with breast cancer pushed her to reexamine the hectic life she was living. Although her tumor was small and her treatment lasted only six weeks, the experience was enough of a shock to put her on a new path. She describes herself as beginning to "seek out a healthier routine, a little introspection, and the time to do my own writing." [20] I could describe the changes in my own life in the exact same words.

I don't want to pretend that changing my life was simple, even after I realized what I wanted to do. After my cancer treatment was over, I spent months wanting to write but feeling guilty about taking time away from Jay's and my business. One day he said he wanted me to do it. He said it was obvious that it was very important to me, and perhaps if I wrote the book I'd been thinking about, it would be important to others as well. He offered to answer all the morning phone calls while I wrote. He would handle what he could and tell people I would call back in the afternoon about the rest. I felt incredibly lucky, and loved, and suddenly free, for the first time in years, to be me.

I know Jay is very special, but I don't think it's unusual for people who love you to support you in doing what's important to you—once you decide what that is. When you find the confidence to believe in yourself, it shows, and the people around you respond. Suddenly things you never thought possible, are possible.

Where Will You Go from Here?

If you are facing cancer, now is a good time to look at your life and set new goals. Nothing clears your vision like confronting your own mortality. Look at your past, look at your present, and decide if the person you are now is the one you want to be for the rest of your life. If not, what can you do to become that person? Some women emerging from breast cancer have taken the major step of quitting their jobs to start the businesses or pursue the careers they always really wanted. Some just reduced the hours or number of days they work to make time for pursuits close to their hearts. Others have kept their full-time jobs but become involved in social, political, or service activities that give them the feeling of fulfillment they had been lacking. Some women simply streamline their lives, dropping activities they were doing out of a sense of obligation to make more time for what they really enjoy. Give yourself some time to change; nobody does it all at once. Think about the first step you want to take, and start planning to take it.

In thinking about all the things you want to live for far into the future, don't underestimate the attraction of ordinary pleasures. We all have leisure-time activities we enjoy doing and look forward to with great anticipation. At first glance, they may not seem terribly important in the overall scheme of life. Perhaps you think of them more as self-indulgence than worthwhile pursuits, that given the seriousness of your situation, they are the first things you should give up. Don't. Any activities that make you happy are important, and they can add significantly to your list of things worth living for. You may be determined to live more usefully in the future, but you can't spend all your time pursuing lofty goals, fighting poverty or injustice, teaching children, comforting the sick, or creating great art. Sometimes you have to indulge in activities for the sheer pleasure they give. If you love to play soccer or go to the movies, read romance novels or build things in your basement workshop, that's an important part of who you are. If the thought of no longer being able to indulge in your favorite activity makes you sad, that's good. It's one more reason you have for regaining your health and getting back to a normal life.

It's especially good if you have annual events you look forward to year after year, like the Super Bowl or an annual family reunion, or if you have things you're waiting anxiously for, like your favorite author's next novel. Think about how great it's going to be and how terrible you would feel to miss it. Whether your passion is music or sports, good restaurants or travel, art or cars—whatever it is, the pleasure it brings to your life is a positive, powerful reason to get healthy and stay healthy. Don't belittle it.

In thinking about the activities you like and want to keep on doing, don't tell yourself you'll pick them up again after you're well. You need them right now, during your medical crisis. I don't know where so many of us got the idea that people who are sick, even if they are not bedridden or in pain, are supposed to stop having fun and just concentrate on their health problems. Having fun is great medicine. It doesn't divert energy from getting well, it adds energy to your body and your life.

So don't sit at home. Call your friends. Go out and do the things you've been wanting to do. One of the positive things I discovered about having cancer is that it gives you a tremendous social advantage. Everyone figures you may be nearing the end, even if you're not, so all your friends want to indulge you. When people are so anxious to make you happy, it would be cruel to deprive them of the opportunity. When someone offers to take you out, or spend time doing what you like to do, learn, as I did, to say, "Yes, thank you."

If there's something you want, now's the time to ask for it. An afternoon at the museum. A walk on the beach. That record album or book you've been wanting to borrow. The recipe a friend has been reluctant to share. Nobody feels good about saying no to someone with cancer. All right, it's a little mischievous, but what's wrong with that? Anyhow, you can always make it up to them later. It will tickle you to get whatever you want for once in your life, and the fun you get out of both the asking and the receiving will be good for your health.

I found I didn't even have to ask for favors most of the time; friends just volunteered. One offered to send me free passes to the Museum of Modern Art, where she is a member, and another took an afternoon off to spend there with me on the day before my surgery. A few days after I got home from the hospital, a live concert tape a musician friend had been promising me for months suddenly showed up at my door. The nice thing was, everyone seemed glad to be able to do something for me, so it was a plus for all of us. The good feelings all around kept my spirits high during what could have been a depressing time. I'm sure they also had a positive effect on my health.

Hang on to Your Identity

It's important to know what's important to you.

I forget most of my dreams as soon as I open my eyes in the morning. Every once in a while, though, I have a Dream with a capital D. They seem to come when something major needs changing in my life. They are far more vivid than my usual dreams, and don't fade away when I wake up. Over the years I have learned to take my big-D dreams seriously, because they obviously come from a part of me that is wiser than any part I have access to when I'm awake. They show me how I'm feeling at times when I'm too caught up in the turmoil of everyday life to see it clearly....

In my big-D dreams I'm almost always in my car. I realized after a few of these dreams that the car is my dream symbol for my life. I'm in my car and something is happening. In one dream, about fifteen years ago, my mother was beside me in the front seat and I ordered her into the back. In another dream, during a particularly difficult time, the car was careening down a hill and I couldn't slow it down. In the dream I had early in my breast cancer ordeal, the car was not out of control, it was simply not under my control. It was going in directions I was not steering. I couldn't make it go where I wanted, and I couldn't get out.

I woke from that dream aware that my life had slipped out of my control. Not because I was sick and might die, but because I was suddenly in a world I didn't understand, where there was no way, and in fact no need, for me to make decisions. I was being steered along from one test to the next, unable to see beyond the next corner. I was moving through a medical maze that was familiar enough to the people telling me which way to go, but was a complete mystery to me. I didn't know where I was headed or what I would find when I got there. I felt completely unable to decide, or even to influence, my own fate.

I sat up in bed, thinking about the dream and what it meant. I knew that since the doctors were still trying to find out if I had cancer or not, there wasn't much for me to do but go along with the process they were putting me through. Once they and I knew, however, I wanted back control of my life. I didn't want major decisions about my future being made by anyone but me.

I have always been fiercely independent, and I know I am more resistant than most people to being told what to do. Still, I think it is important for any woman facing a medical crisis to stop early on and think about how much say you are going to have in your treatment. If you have breast cancer, someone is going to be making tough decisions. You may decide to hand over to your doctors the power to make those decisions. Some women do—but I hope you won't, not without thinking about it first. Many questions will arise, and the answers are not as straightforward as you may think. There will be important choices to be made. No matter how much you trust your doctors, remember that it is *your* body and *your* future that are in jeopardy. *You* are the one who will undergo surgery or radiation. *You* will be the one who suffers the side effects of drugs, chemotherapy, or reconstruction. Not your doctor—*you*. Although it is certainly true that your doctor knows more about cancer than you do, you know more about your own body and about what's important in your life.

First You Have to Know Yourself

During my months of testing, I dug as deep as I could into my feelings, trying to discover what I really cared about. The conclusions I reached weren't earthshaking. They were pretty obvious, really, except that I had never bothered to articulate them before. The thing I cared about most was staying alive. No surprise there. To achieve that goal, I was determined to get the best medical care I could. After that, I just wanted to get the whole cancer ordeal over with as soon as possible and get back to my normal life.

As I thought about what getting back to normal meant to me, I realized it didn't necessarily mean that my body had to be the same. I wanted to go on feeling strong and healthy; whether I did it with one breast or two didn't really matter. It was my life, not my body, that I wanted to get back to the way it was.

I realized, too, how very important it was to me to be treated as an individual. I didn't like the feeling that as far as the hospital was concerned I was, if not a number, something of a statistic. I was another woman with a suspicious lump in her breast being put through the routine that every woman with a suspicious lump in her breast goes through.

All of the medical professionals I dealt with—doctors, nurses, technicians, and receptionists—were kind, but they were also hurried and impersonal. Now, looking back, I can see that they didn't have much choice. Our medical system is organized to treat a great many sick people as efficiently as possible, not to cater to individuals. Protocols have been established for handling patients with life-threatening conditions like breast cancer; systems are in place, and both patients and professionals are expected to fit themselves into the proper roles. If that leaves you feeling like the proverbial square peg in a round hole, nobody but you even has the time to notice.

The people who work in this complex and overburdened system have learned to sort patients into categories, each of which is characterized by a set of assumptions and suitable treatments. When patients' symptoms and attitudes fit the assumptions of the category they are put in, the system works pretty well. When someone comes along who doesn't fit, everyone gets thrown for a loop.

I got my first inkling of this when Dr. S. tried to "stage" my cancer. Staging is another word for categorizing cancer patients. The first thing a doctor looks at to decide the stage of a cancer is the size of the lump. A lump that is less than 2 centimeters in diameter falls into stage 1, a category with a pretty good prognosis, so long as the underarm lymph nodes don't show any traces of cancer. A lump that is more than 2 centimeters is stage 2, a not-so-good category, regardless of the state of the lymph nodes. The rules for staging are pretty straightforward. The experts who established them evidently didn't add a footnote to cover variations such as two lumps in the same breast.

Dr. S. wasn't sure how to stage me. I had two side-by-side lumps, each about 1.5 centimeters. He told me that if he considered them separately, I was stage 1. If he added them together, I was stage 2. There were evidently no guidelines to cover the aberrant behavior of my cancer. The doctor was on his own; I had messed up the system. He finally decided to consider the tumors separately, which made me stage 1, and gave me a much better chance of surviving than if he had decided to add them together. It seemed to me that my chance of survival would not be affected in the least by the label he attached to my cancer. Treatment recommendations, however, are affected, so staging is not to be taken lightly.

Medical Care Is Based on Generalizations

I didn't fit the psychological and emotional assumptions about women with breast cancer any better than I fit the physical guidelines. For one thing, I have an aversion to taking drugs. I don't trust them to limit their actions to what they are meant to do inside my body and nothing else. I don't even take aspirin for a headache unless I am in pretty severe pain. But since I was a breast surgery patient, it was assumed I would want painkillers.

Shortly after I was wheeled into my room after my mastectomy, someone hooked a morphine delivery system into the intravenous tube in my arm and showed me which button to push whenever I wanted a dose. It is a nifty new system that allows patients to get quick relief when they need it, and reportedly results in patients taking less drugs than under the old medication-according-to-a-schedule system.

What no one seemed to notice was that I didn't have any pain—none at all. I did have curiosity, though—no doubt left over from my younger, more experimental days. I lay there, alone in my room, the morphine button by my side, wondering what a hit would feel like and whether it would get me high. After a short internal debate on the ethics of the situation, I pushed the button, twice. The effect was hardly noticeable (I guess because there was no pain to kill), so I left the button alone after that. Every few hours a nurse would come in to record the amount of morphine I had taken. She would stare at the machine for a few moments and then walk out. Eventually someone came and took the morphine away.

The day after the operation I felt fine and was anxious to go home. But wait—hospital procedures said I needed pain pills to take along. Without consulting me, a prescription was sent to the pharmacy downstairs, and I had to wait a seemingly interminable time for the pills to arrive, before the doctor on duty would release me. When I got home I put the bottle of pills in the linen closet; I never took a single one. I was more than a little annoyed when a bill for them came in the mail.

A week after surgery, I went back to have my staples removed. The surgeon who removed them (Dr. S. was on vacation) saw that the flesh around them was red and puffy, and said I should take antibiotics. Here we go again, I thought, more unnecessary drugs. This time I spoke up. I said my body was probably just trying to get rid of the staples and that I'd be fine once they were out. The surgeon looked at me thoughtfully and then, to my amazement, agreed that I might be right. Instead of insisting that I take the antibiotics, he gave me a prescription I could fill if I felt I needed them. It sat on my desk for several weeks before I threw it away.

Bucking Longstanding Attitudes

After that small victory, I began asserting myself more and more, refusing to take medication or advice that didn't make sense to me. I grew increasingly impatient with doctors who assumed they knew what I was feeling, both physically and emotionally. I know I startled some of them by my stubbornness and my determination to make my own decisions. Dr. S. commented one day that I was very different from most of his female patients. I wondered about that. Most of the women I know are strong and sensible, not only capable of making serious decisions but used to doing so for both themselves and others. Do they really let go so easily when a disease like breast cancer strikes? Do they shrink into obedient silence just when they have everything to fight for? Evidently many do. I've spent a good deal of time trying to figure out why.

Obviously, when you discover you have breast cancer you are likely to be scared and confused, at least at first. More significant, though, are the attitudes you encounter—especially inside the hospital—from all the people who assume you are overwhelmed by your situation, are incapable of understanding highly sophisticated medical treatments, and want nothing so much as to be told what to do. At times, those assumptions might not be far from the truth. There is a part of any sick person that wants to pass the burden of a cure on to someone else, to lie back and be miraculously rescued. Given the patriarchal structure of our medical system and our society's longstanding attitudes toward women, it's not surprising if a woman with breast cancer feels that way.

As Americans, we all grew up surrounded by romantic stories of the helpless female and the powerful, heroic male. The images are ubiquitous and inescapable in our cultural mythology. The most obvious is the archetypal damsel in distress, tied to the railroad tracks, with a locomotive bearing down on her and her heroic rescuer arriving in the nick of time to whisk her out of harm's way. Then there's the brave knight on horseback fighting for his lady. The handsome prince breaking the curse on Sleeping Beauty with a kiss or snatching Cinderella from a life of loveless drudgery. The rugged cowboy saving the frightened frontier woman from a gang of bad guys. The tough cop, the nervy private detective. And, of course, the smart, dedicated, highly skilled doctor.

Like so many of the women she has read about and seen on-screen, the woman with breast cancer knows she is in serious danger and feels unable to save herself. Suddenly she is the helpless maiden, tied to the tracks, with the cancer train bearing down on her. The oncologist or surgeon fits easily into the role of heroic rescuer. The scenario feels so familiar, so comforting, that it can be difficult to resist being drawn into it.

Despite their seductive power, the helpless female/heroic male roles would probably not carry over so easily to the real-life medical setting, were they not reinforced there by the mythology of the medical world itself. Modern medical practice is, after all, both strongly male-dominated and drenched in the mystique of the heroic.

It is very important for any woman facing breast cancer to be aware that when you enter the medical realm you are walking into one of the great male strongholds of our culture, and that the higher you go within the system, the more exclusively male it becomes. As a patient who has or may have cancer, you go straight to the top, to the heady areas of surgery and oncology, where male doctors indisputably rule. That is not to say that there are no female surgeons or female oncologists in the American medical system. Of course there are, some of them outstanding and quite well known. But their numbers are small. Most women with breast cancer are treated by men.

Men, Women, and
the Practice of Medicine

◎

Most of us, born in the twentieth century, have always known medical care in its current, specialized, male-dominated form. When we find ourselves in a health crisis, we look to the doctor as a contemporary version of the knight in shining armor, who comes striding to our rescue, armed with miracle drugs and, if necessary, a scalpel, to vanquish any enemy that threatens our well-being. Few of us realize that the practice of medicine was taken over by doctors and masculinized only about 200 years ago. In their eye-opening book *For Her Own Good*, [21] Barbara Ehrenreich and Dierdre English describe how before the Industrial Revolution health care was an integral part of family and community life and was almost entirely the domain of women. Healing practices were based not on scientific research but on intuition, compassion, personal experience, and a wide-ranging, shared knowledge of the healing effects of plants, potions, and loving care. It was a system in many ways less well informed than the one we have today, and in many ways wiser.

In the mid-eighteenth century, when the center of economic life moved from the home to the urban factory, health care too moved out of the family and into the marketplace, out of the hands of women and into the hands of men. Soon formal education (which was mostly denied to women) was established as a requirement for the right to heal the sick, and highly structured medical research began to replace centuries of intuition and shared experience.

Sometime in the mid-nineteenth century, the leaders of the new medical science decided that its most important challenge was explaining every function of the human body in physiochemical terms. In the rational, controlled, male-dominated world of the laboratory, the secrets of health were sought under the microscope rather than in the bodies and minds of the sick. A fascination with cells, molecules, and man-made drugs, for better or worse, became the driving force in health care.

By the twentieth century, medicine had become the highly respected, stubbornly scientific, and overwhelmingly male profession we know today. Within its powerful institutions researchers swept aside the observations and reported experiences of patients, labeling them "nonscientific" and therefore irrelevant. "Anecdotal evidence," the scientists' name for patients' personal stories, became a pejorative term. A fact was real only if it could be demonstrated in controlled studies, preferably performed in a laboratory, and not just once, but several times.

What does all this mean to a woman diagnosed with breast cancer today? It means that when you walk into your doctor's office or hospital, you are walking into the hallowed, male-dominated halls of science, where you should not expect your common sense, intuition, or experience to carry much weight. This does not mean you should check them at the door. On the contrary, you will need them to evaluate all the "facts" and advice you are going to hear so that you can decide what makes sense for you and what doesn't.

The era of the family doctor, when doctors at least made house calls and saw their patients in the context of their lives, is now gone. In most places today a doctor is so completely outside of the lives of his patients, and so pressed for time, that he has little choice but to judge their conditions by the measures and predictions—generalizations really—that come from researchers' laboratories. The medical system allows for nothing else.

We, however, can buck the system, if we are willing to speak up. We can insist that our doctors see us as people. We can point out when their assumptions about us are wrong, and their suggested treatments inappropriate. Once, when Dr. S. finally backed off from a recommendation I had repeatedly refused to accept, he said, "Well, I don't know you. How could I?" I appreciated that he had made a big concession, setting aside his scientific formula long enough to concede that perhaps I knew better what was right for me.

Be a Smart "Shopper"

If you are going to evaluate and decide among the treatments that are suggested for you, it helps to have some understanding not only of the treatments themselves, but of the general approach of the research industry that has developed them. That industry has two parts—the scientists who search for basic understanding and effective treatments, and the companies, government agencies, and philanthropic groups and individuals who fund and oversee the research.

One of the first and most upsetting things I found out when I began looking into the testing aspect of medical research is that women have been systematically excluded from some of the most basic studies. The measure of success for drug testing is often the consistency and reproducibility of the results. Many researchers find women's bodies too changeable, too complicated, and too unpredictable for their scientific purposes. As many of us know, even one of a woman's most regular functions—her monthly period—can be thrown off by changes of habit or location, by excitement or upsets. Baffled as to how to compensate for the cyclical changes in women's bodies (to say nothing of the serendipitous ones), many researchers have simply left women out of their studies. Most major scientific research—including the famous study that decided aspirin can reduce the incidence of second heart attacks, influential studies on cholesterol and on smoking, and virtually all studies on pain and pain relief—has been conducted exclusively on men. [22] Nobody knows whether the conclusions drawn from these studies also apply to women. Doctors apply the "knowledge" that the studies have produced to women anyway, because it's science, and it's all the "acceptable" data they have to go on.

Of course, some studies have focused on women—breast cancer studies, for instance. Mostly, the results show that scientists are confounded. After decades of research—admittedly, limited research with limited funding—we don't even have a dependable method of detecting a cancer that's been growing in a woman's breast for ten years or more. Mammography, the best method we have so far, produces a high percentage of false positive and false negative results. [23] The vast majority of breast tumors are still discovered by women themselves or their lovers.

It appears at first glance that the most useful breast cancer information researchers have provided us is in the area of "risk factors." You've probably read in newspapers or seen on TV enthusiastic reports that scientists have identified the "breast cancer gene." Unfortunately, their discovery doesn't help women who already have the disease. It's even more disappointing that this knowledge doesn't do much to predict who will get breast cancer either, since only about 5 percent of diagnosed cases have a genetic link, and women who have the gene do not necessarily get cancer. [24]

Scientists, of course, have also been looking for causes of the nearly 95 percent of breast cancer cases that are not genetic, and they have come up with a culprit: estrogen. Researchers have decided that the more estrogen a woman has in her body during her lifetime, the greater her chance of getting breast cancer. [25] Now, even we laywomen know that estrogen is the underlying source of our femaleness, the big-honcho hormone that controls everything that makes a woman a woman. Reduced to its essence, what the scientists are telling us is that being a woman puts you at risk for breast cancer. I guess that's true. It's also true that breathing puts you at risk for lung cancer, if you do it where there is cigarette smoke, asbestos, or some other carcinogen in the air.

Researchers have developed the somewhat bizarre premise that "exposure" to our own estrogen is dangerous (as if someone can be exposed to what is most basic in herself). From there, they have gone on to implicate the many factors of a woman's life that indicate her body has a high estrogen level. They say she is in danger if she starts menstruating early, stops menstruating late, starts having children late or has too few or none, doesn't breast-feed, and on and on. Basically, the woman of past centuries—who began menstruating in her mid-teens, married soon thereafter, and was either pregnant or breast-feeding, or both, until menopause—is the medical ideal. Science seems to be telling us that the changes women have managed to make in our lives (we call it progress) have backfired, and put us all at risk.

Once researchers have a theory that makes sense to them, they set out to test that theory, and sometimes slip into a kind of tunnel vision. Assuming that more estrogen causes more breast cancer, they look for conditions known to result from strong supplies of estrogen, such as dense bones, then look for a higher incidence of cancer in women who have them. If they find it, as indeed one study did, they offer it to us as yet another proof that having a healthy supply of estrogen puts us at risk. If you look beyond the publicized results of the research, however, you sometimes find more interesting facts.

Reading about the dense bones research, for instance, I found that the statistics emerged from a health study that followed a group of Massachusetts women for 50 years. [26] Of the 1,373 women, 91 developed breast cancer. That's 6.6 percent, or 1 in 15. It occurred to me that rather than an indictment of estrogen, the study could be cited as a demonstration that the breast cancer risk statistic we have all been frightened by—the ominous one in eight—is off by nearly 100 percent.

Since the overall incidence of breast cancer was not what the researchers were looking for, however, they don't seem to have noticed.

I'm uncomfortable with all the attention being paid to the estrogen theory of breast cancer, mostly for two reasons. First, it sidesteps the most important questions. What I want to know, as with any other disease, is not who is susceptible to breast cancer, but what causes it, and how do we stop it? If we can remove the cause, it will no longer matter who is susceptible. Second, since some 75 percent of women who get breast cancer don't have any of the risk factors researchers have identified, [27] I find it hard to understand why these even qualify as major risk factors, or why so much time and money is being spent on pursuing them.

Who Decides What's Good for Us?

More alarming to me than the scientists' approach to medical research is the way that research is financed. Today many of the most important studies are paid for by the companies that will manufacture and profit from the drugs and techniques being tested. I believe drug companies want to find treatments that are effective, but I also believe they focus their attention on developing treatments that are patentable and profitable. As patients, we need to understand that health care in America is big business. The drugs that are best for a pharmaceutical company's bottom line may or may not also be best for us. It is naive to think our health is the only thing on a drug company's mind.

Many of us unquestioningly trust the drugs prescribed for us because we believe they are all carefully tested, evaluated, and monitored by the government. In fact, government-sponsored research has declined in the past two decades, and drug companies have spent huge amounts on lobbying efforts to reduce the power of government regulation. According to Public Citizen, a consumer watchdog group founded by Ralph Nader, between 1992 and 1996 conservative think tanks spearheading a movement to curb the FDA's regulatory powers received at least $3.5 million from drug and tobacco companies, who want to see the approval process, as well as research, in the hands of private companies. [28]

The big drug companies are also putting lots of money into advertising, which used to be aimed at doctors but lately has shifted focus to reach a more mainstream audience. Ubiquitous advertising is making drugs seem like a natural element of everyday life and is gradually erasing our resistance to them.

In her book *The Beauty Myth*, [29] Naomi Wolf suggests that American women's self-images have been so weakened by the relentless assault of advertising and popular culture that we have been rendered incapable of resisting anything advertisers claim will improve our images or our lives. I rebel at the thought, and want to prove her wrong, but deep inside I fear that, in many cases, she is right. We may be smart consumers when we shop for clothes or cars or gifts for those we love, but when it comes to the appearance and health of our bodies, we sometimes become the damsel in distress—frightened, desperate, and too dazzled by anyone who comes to our rescue to question his methods. We need to learn to be as careful in evaluating health-care products as we are in sizing up other consumer products.

As Norman Cousins points out in *Anatomy of an Illness*, "the history of medicine is replete with accounts of drugs and modes of treatment that were in use for many years before it was recognized that they did more harm than good." [30] He uses the example of doctors for centuries bleeding patients for virtually every illness. In our own time, there has been a years-long investigation of the violent psychological side effects of the widely prescribed sleeping pill Halcion®, and a ban on the popular allergy drug Seldane®, [31] which has been linked to potentially fatal heart problems. In September 1996 a study of a heart-monitoring procedure called right-heart catheterization, in use for 25 years, disclosed that it increased the death rate of patients by 21 percent.[32] There are countless other examples of commonly prescribed drugs and medical procedures that have turned out to be useless or worse.

I do not mean to say that current breast cancer treatments are harmful, but none has been shown to be completely effective, all are controversial in one way or another, and all come with potentially serious side effects. Some, though widely used, are still being tested. It would be nice to have a surefire cure that works for everyone, but so far we don't.

Ultimately, it's up to you decide what treatment you will undergo. To make the best choice, think about which of the treatments offered to you best fits you as an individual. Be sure your doctors know what your particular concerns are, especially if one form of treatment is more frightening to you, for some reason, than another. Perhaps a different approach will be just as effective. With drugs, even after treatment is under way you can change your mind if you decide what you chose is wrong for you.

In a moving and insightful article entitled "My Life with Cancer" in the Spring 1997 Ms. magazine, writer Patricia Jones Bacchus explains why she decided to discontinue her chemotherapy regime partway through. "I don't bicker with the fact that I need chemotherapy," she writes, "I simply contest the drugs they were giving me. It is a fact, acknowledged by the doctors, that one of the drugs I received is toxic to the heart, and I have experienced irregular and increased heartbeats. It is also an acknowledged fact that one of the other drugs put me at risk for leukemia as well as lymphoma....Today, they know the risks associated with these drugs, yet they did not tell me. Everything I know about these risks I discovered through my own research. Be that as it may, if I were to finish the treatment only to end up with heart failure, or leukemia, or lymphoma, it would be no consolation whatsoever to my husband, my daughter, or my mother to know that I didn't die of breast cancer."

Later, Bacchus found a different oncologist and started treatment anew with different drugs. "His opinion was thoughtful and thoroughly explained. The most important thing he did for me, though, was listen to me, and respect both my fears and wishes. And he also told me honestly about the risk of other cancers with these drugs. I have accepted these risks, and I have no complaints or second thoughts."

Ask questions, do as much reading on your own as you can, listen to the information and advice your doctors give you, then apply your own good sense. Don't worry. If you are realistic and thoughtful and clear as to what is important to you, you will make good choices.

Today doctors are coming to realize what the healers of past centuries knew very well: there are many factors that influence the effectiveness of a treatment, and the cooperation and involvement of the patient rank high among them. A breast cancer specialist I heard speak at a women's health conference said her statistics show the treatment a woman chooses is actually less important than the fact that she has made the choice. Patients who choose their treatment, she said, do better than those who have treatments thrust on them, regardless of what treatment they choose.

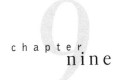
Teach—and Understand— Your Doctors

Insist on a doctor you trust.

While it is generally true that doctors don't see their patients as individuals, it is also true that most patients don't see their doctors as individuals. As health care has become more standardized and more controlled by people other than doctors themselves, the doctor-patient relationship has become increasingly impersonal, a situation which is harmful to both doctor and patient. We must not accept the deterioration of this important alliance as just one more casualty of modern life....

As we rush through our hectic days, how many of the people we interact with do we really get to know, and how many do we allow to know us? Does your car mechanic have a family? Where is your mailman from? What does your child's teacher do during summer vacation? Could any of these people answer the same questions about you?

When I was young I had an uncle who was a mailman in White Plains, New York. The people on his route loved him because he chatted with them as he delivered their mail and they got to know each other. Occasionally they would tell him about small problems they had—a broken toaster is one I remember—and he would take a few minutes from his rounds to see if he could help. I don't think there are many mailmen like my Uncle Tom anymore. I don't think we and the people who perform services for us take the time to think about each other as people anymore.

We live in a fast-paced, crowded, complicated world where the sense of community, and the reality of community, have been fading for years. Some of us actually feel that we know the people we see on television better than we know the people in our everyday lives. It is, of course, an illusion. We don't know the people we see on television, and they certainly don't know us. The lives we watch them leading are not real; they are performances.

Mass communication, while entertaining us, has blurred the lines between real and fantasized relationships. It has taught us to imagine ourselves connected to others because we see them and hear them, without ever having to communicate with them, or, as we feel increasingly insecure, without having to expose ourselves to them. In many ways our own lives have become performances. We interact with most people on a superficial level, sharing just enough time and conversation to accomplish what we need to get done. We show only the parts of ourselves we want others to see, and hide the real, deep feelings—the fears, hopes, and desires—that motivate so much of what we do. We think it doesn't matter, and in many parts of our lives, perhaps it doesn't.

Then we get sick, and we go to see a doctor. For many of us, the experience is no different from the hundreds of other interactions that make up our lives. We sit in a sterile examining room and watch the doctor's face as he searches our chart and our body for the cause of our illness. We answer his questions, telling him just what he needs to know about us. He tells us nothing about himself. What should be one of the most intimate exchanges between people, an honest and open discussion between doctor and patient, is instead a cold and distant survey of symptoms.

For a patient worried that she may have breast cancer, such a relationship—or nonrelationship—can add to feelings of bewilderment and helplessness. When you are facing a serious disease, you need a doctor who can boost your confidence and optimism as well as treat your symptoms. You need a doctor you can talk to, one who will talk to you, and will listen. Even in this age of high technology and managed health care, it is every patient's right, and responsibility, to seek such a doctor.

So, how do you do it?

Finding the Right Doctor for You

First, it is important to know that there are lots of good doctors. You can find one you like and trust if you make the effort. No one else can do this for you. Only you can decide who feels right to you. The doctor your friend or mother or cousin loves may not be the doctor for you.

Second, be clear in your own mind as to what you want and can reasonably expect from a doctor. Keep reminding yourself that doctors are people, just like you and me. Most sincerely want to help their patients, but their knowledge and their tools have limits. The doctor-as-god mindset, so prevalent in my parents' generation, is at best unwise, at worst downright dangerous. It burdens doctors with too much responsibility for other people's lives and makes patients feel they have no control or influence over their situation.

I know that when you are in an urgent predicament, as you are when a possible tumor has been detected in your breast, you don't feel that you have a lot of time for shopping around. Nevertheless, it is terribly important to find a doctor you feel comfortable with. Perhaps you will click with the first specialist you see. If you do, heave a sigh of relief and start building your relationship with him or her. If, on the other hand, the first doctor you see is uncommunicative or makes you uncomfortable in any serious way, say you want a second opinion and go consult someone else.

Of all the good feelings you would like to have toward the doctor who is going to help you through your health crisis, trust is perhaps the most important. Studies have shown that patients who trust their doctors are more likely to recover from their illnesses. I think it stands to reason that having confidence in your doctor will make you feel calmer and more optimistic, both of which are positive forces in recovery and healing.

If you're going to have surgery, as most breast cancer patients do, it's vital that you find a surgeon you feel comfortable with. Going under the knife is never a happy prospect, so it's essential, if you're going to go into it calmly, that you feel you've got the best surgeon around. Talk to as many as it takes to find one you're willing to have cut into you.

Look for a surgeon who is known for his skill and has had lots of practice in the particular operation you're facing. Ask people you know for recommendations of surgeons they have used and liked. When you go to consult a surgeon, ask how many times he has done this particular operation and how his patients have fared. Remember that an interview with a surgeon is not just an opportunity for him to find out about you. While he is evaluating your condition, you should be evaluating him. You can't tell everything about a doctor, but you can get a feeling for what he's like.

Personality is not as important as training, experience, and skill, but it does matter. You know what kinds of people make you feel positive and energetic. Look for a surgeon who is like that. You are going to need all the positive energy you can muster to heal quickly after your surgery. One reason I switched from Dr. R., a very nice man, was that I didn't think his soft-spoken, gentle manner was going to propel me back onto my feet. I wanted a doctor with vigorous energy that would help to push me forward. Both Dr. R. and Dr. S. are good surgeons. Dr. S. just fit better with my own personality. Don't underestimate the subtle effects that someone else's personality can have on you, especially when that someone is there to help you pull through a crisis.

If you're not sure what kind of person will make you feel most comfortable, think about what kinds of things cheer you up when you are feeling down or worried. Do you long for a quiet walk in the woods? I like peaceful places when I'm feeling good, but when I'm upset or worried I'm not drawn to serenity. I go to the ocean to watch the waves crashing against the shore. I like to feel their power. I also lose interest in slow, sensitive music during difficult times. When I need my spirits lifted, I put on loud rock 'n' roll, the stronger and more driving the beat, the better. These things may not appear to be related to your choice of doctor, but I think they are important clues to what kind of energy lifts your spirits. All other things being equal, you'll do better with a doctor who fits your personal style. (If the technical abilities of doctors you're comparing aren't equal, by all means select for skill and reputation.)

Since you and your doctor will be working together to overcome your cancer, you should size him up as you would anyone you're going to work closely with. Be absolutely sure you can communicate easily. You shouldn't have to learn a foreign language to talk with your doctor. Every professional specialty, from computer programming to fashion design, has its own vocabulary, and medicine's is one of the most multisyllabic and foreign-sounding. But doctors deal with ordinary people every day; they know how to speak English. If a doctor insists on battering you with jargon, look elsewhere, until you find someone who is more interested in communicating with you than impressing or intimidating you.

Even more important than finding a doctor who speaks clearly is finding one who listens. Too many doctors don't listen to patients or don't take what their patients, especially their female patients, say very seriously. They are used to getting most of their information from other doctors—in medical journals, at seminars, or in personal conversations. They put a lot of trust in published statistics and the conventional wisdom that is dispensed at meetings and conventions. The broad observations and conclusions that are circulated among them eventually take on the appearance of absolute truth and then, too often, get applied to individual patients whether they fit or not. If you don't want to receive cookie-cutter treatment, there will be occasions when you're going to have to speak up. Make sure you've got a doctor who will listen.

Patient to Doctor = Person to Person

If you've always looked up to doctors, it may be hard to start seeing them as your equals. Most of us have an image of doctors as somehow bigger than us—more educated, more skilled, richer, more respected, and perhaps more deserving of respect. They are pretty high up in our cultural pantheon of heroes. These attitudes, and the whole structure of the medical system, make it hard for us to see that doctors are people, just like us, and that the ideal doctor-patient relationship is a partnership.

A doctor needs to know a lot about two things to be effective in helping you. He needs to know about the disease or condition you are suffering from, and he needs to know about your body. If he is well trained, smart, and experienced, he probably knows enough about your disease. But what does he know about your body? At the start of your relationship, nothing. Bodies are different. They have different levels of energy. Some heal quickly, others slowly. Some have a high tolerance for drugs, others have a low tolerance. Some need lots of sleep, others need lots of exercise. Some are subject to headaches, others to stomach upset, others to skin problems. You know your body. When you walk into a doctor's office you bring with you half the information he needs to do his job well.

You also bring an essential healing tool that no doctor can provide—your attitude. If you enter the relationship with optimism, faith, and a determination to get well, your doctor will find your body's natural healing mechanisms ready to respond to his efforts. If you come with fear, resentment, and pessimism, your doctor will have to overcome the obstacles you unconsciously throw in his path, in addition to your disease. The combination may be too powerful. Add your knowledge of your body and a positive attitude to your doctor's knowledge of disease and available treatments, and you've got a working whole, a partnership with good prospects for success.

The wonderful thing about a good partnership is that it produces a level of results neither individual could accomplish alone. I have learned that lesson through work relationships, but I think it applies in every area of our lives. As an editor, I have worked with a number of graphic designers. My favorite, and the one with whom I turned out the best projects, has a stunning visual sense, but he sometimes brought me design ideas I felt would make a book harder to read. I would reject part of a design and then realize that while the problem was glaring to me, it was news to him. Each of us saw clearly what we wanted to accomplish, but needed to learn what was important to the other. Despite our conflicts, we always made a great effort to cooperate, and even when we got frustrated we kept on communicating. We knew that if we could make the design and editorial content fit each other, we would both win. If not, we would both have failed.

In a medical setting, if the treatment works and is right for the patient, both doctor and patient win. If the treatment stops the disease but upsets the psychological and emotional functioning of the patient, does the doctor win and the patient lose? No, they both lose. The doctor loses because he has treated the disease but not the patient. If I had let Dr. S. talk me into reconstructive breast surgery, I have no doubt I would have been miserable, scarred emotionally as well as physically. If I had agreed to take the hormonal drug tamoxifen, recommended by the oncologist I consulted, I would have been terrified every day that I was doing something harmful to my body. My doctors had no way of knowing how I felt until I told them. Every patient has the responsibility of letting your doctor know what is going on in the parts of you he cannot see—your mind and emotions.

Stay on Your Toes

When you start seeing doctors as people rather than members of some higher order, it becomes easier to interact with them. You also begin to see that they have the same strengths and weaknesses as the rest of us, which can be disconcerting. We all want to trust our doctors, and usually we can. I've had enough bad experiences, however, to realize that some doctors should not be trusted. You need to be as watchful of doctors as you are of anyone else who provides you a service, and be ready to fire a doctor who crosses the line.

Of the three doctors I've had negative experiences with, two were dentists. The first was simply incompetent. He was my family dentist when I was a child. I didn't learn until years later that he regularly left decay in the teeth he filled and they continued deteriorating under the fillings. As an adult, I had a dentist I considered quite good. I respected and trusted him until one particular checkup, when he somberly informed me that I needed three root canals and at least two new crowns right away. Each of these urgently needed items was expensive, and I had very little money at the time. I left that appointment stunned and worried. Outside I saw a building permit posted on the wall; my dentist was about to expand his office. Wondering how much his building plans had to do with my sudden need for dental work, I called another dentist and asked for a second opinion. After examining my teeth and a new set of x-rays, he told me I needed one root canal, not three, and that I had a couple of crowns that should be replaced, sometime in the next ten years. I switched dentists.

My third medical misadventure started with a swollen finger. Over the course of a week the swelling got larger, redder, and hotter, until I decided I had to do something about it. I went to the outpatient urgent care department of a nearby hospital. The resident there feared something was seriously wrong and referred me to a specialist, an orthopedic surgeon. The surgeon x-rayed the finger and found that a small section of bone had been eaten away. He was stumped as to what was causing this strange condition and said only exploratory surgery would give him the answer.

At the time I was an enthusiastic guitar student. The surgeon said he would not remove any bone, because that would make it hard for me to play. He thought he could find out what he needed to know from a sample of the surrounding soft tissue. As it turned out, the tissue he removed and sent off to be examined showed nothing wrong. He was completely baffled, and was even more surprised when his follow-up x-rays showed the bone was healing. The hole was not getting any larger, and its edges were becoming smooth. The swelling, redness, and heat were also gone. Whatever had been happening inside my finger, it wasn't happening anymore. The surgeon told me to come back in two weeks for another x-ray.

When I returned to his office he announced that he wanted to operate again, this time to remove a bone sample. I was amazed. "Isn't it healing?" I asked. He said it was. "Then why operate a second time?" He told me he belonged to a doctors group that met once a month over lunch to discuss their most interesting cases. His colleagues were intrigued by my finger and wanted more information. I refused. He looked surprised. I remember thinking this was not a man used to having his patients say no. I told him I didn't care what had caused the problem. I only cared that it was gone. He accepted my decision, but he obviously was not happy that he had been unable to diagnose and treat me. He pulled open his desk drawer, took out some drug company samples of antibiotics, and said he wanted me to take them.

"But isn't the infection gone?" I asked. He said it was. "Then why take antibiotics?" He put the pills back in the drawer. In finally dismissing me from his care, he said he thought my condition had been caused by some anaerobic microorganism that died when he cut the finger open and exposed it to the air. I didn't object to that suggestion, since it seemed to make him feel better, and it didn't cost me anything.

A few weeks later my mother mentioned my strange finger problem to her doctor in Massachusetts. "Does your daughter have psoriasis?" he asked. My mother said I did. Her doctor said he had just read a medical journal article that said psoriasis, generally thought of as a skin condition, can attack bones, actually eating away pieces of them. I think he had probably hit on the answer, but I never called the orthopedic surgeon to tell him. The day he decided his colleagues' curiosity was more important than my finger, he lost my respect.

Actually, of the three doctors I feel mistreated me, the surgeon is the one I have some mixed feelings about. It is easy to condemn a doctor who damages his patients through incompetence, and one who would perform unnecessary operations in order to finance an expansion of his office. It is harder to write off a desire for medical knowledge. Doctors do, after all, learn about diseases, and about drugs as well, by seeing what they do to people. It is a conflict built into the practice of medicine. As patients, we need to be aware of this conflict, and always be clear as to our own interests.

The Patient-versus-Science Conflict

When you are ill, it's your health that should be on your doctor's mind, not the advancement of science. This seems such an obvious point that it shouldn't even need saying. And yet there are many, many stories of patients being used for research without their knowledge or consent.

Some instances seem very minor, unless you are the one being used. A few years ago my mother, who was in her late 70s at the time, was in the hospital with an ailment the doctors could not figure out.

When I called her one day she was in tears. Her own doctor had said she was well enough to go home, but the staff doctors at the hospital were keeping her there because they were still curious and wanted to do more tests. She was exhausted and frightened. Furious, I called her doctor, who didn't know the hospital had delayed her release. He called immediately and told them to send her home.

My mother's experience was nothing compared to that of many people who have been used deliberately and outrageously to satisfy medical curiosity. In April 1997 President Clinton officially apologized to the survivors of the so-called Tuskegee Study, conducted from 1932 to 1972, in which the U.S. Public Health Service withheld treatment from 399 black men with syphilis because doctors wanted to study how the disease spreads and kills. During that same period and on into the 1980s, a number of tests were conducted on unsuspecting patients to give doctors information about the effects of radiation. [33]

The public is always outraged when such studies are exposed, but the practice goes on nonetheless. In December 1996, the Cleveland *Plain Dealer* obtained a batch of FDA files under the Freedom of Information Act. The files revealed that in checking up on more than 4,000 "researchers testing new drugs on humans, the FDA cited more than 53 percent for failing to fully disclose the experimental nature of their work." [34] In other words, the patients receiving the drugs did not know that those drugs were experimental. Failure to disclose that a drug, or any medical procedure, is experimental has been illegal since the end of World War II.

As patients, we have the right to know if a drug or other treatment recommended for us is experimental, or if tests performed on us are for our benefit or for the sake of research. If you have doubts about whether your doctor is telling you everything, speak up. The best way to get the truth is often simply to ask.

In addition to situations in which patients don't know they are being used as experimental subjects, there has been serious concern about studies in which volunteers are not fully informed of the dangers they may face as a result of tests they agree to participate in. One study that has been strongly criticized is the recently completed test of the breast cancer drug tamoxifen. More than 13,000 healthy but "high risk" female volunteers took the drug for five years to see if it would lower their susceptibility. In October 1992, several U.S. Congressional committees concluded that many of the participating women were given overly optimistic views of the drug's potential benefits, and were not given crucial information about its risks. Among numerous other serious side effects, tamoxifen can cause potentially fatal blood clots and a particularly virulent form of uterine cancer. In addition to voicing concern about participants being fully informed, the committee questioned whether it is ethical in the first place to subject healthy women to such dangers. The testing was stopped for a short time, then resumed. In February 1996, the International Agency for Research on Cancer, a division of the World Health Organization, classified tamoxifen as a Group 1 carcinogen. (Group 1 means the Agency has no doubt of its carcinogenic effects.) American researchers claimed that this declaration was not sufficient reason to discontinue the study. [35]

When the oncologist I consulted recommended that I take tamoxifen following my mastectomy, he did not mention that it could cause uterine cancer, the side effect that concerned me most. Neither did Dr. S., who does not recommend follow-up therapies but seemed to assume I would take the drug, as millions of women who have had breast cancer already do. (Tamoxifen is one of the most widely prescribed drugs in the world.) Nor did either doctor mention to me that while tamoxifen had shown some effectiveness in postmenopausal women, it had not been proven helpful for premenopausal women, of which I was and still am one. I decided against taking the drug.

How can these doctors be so seemingly casual about recommending dangerous, unproven drugs? Are they, like the doctors in the orthopedic surgeon's lunch group, more interested in advancing their knowledge than in the welfare of their patients? I don't think that's what's going on. I believe, rather, that many patients are getting caught between two very different views of health care—the patient's and the doctor's—and that both doctors and patients need to understand the differences if we are going to work effectively as partners.

Two Different Worlds

I realized at some point during my breast cancer treatment that a doctor's world is very different from the average person's. It took a while for this to dawn on me, but when it did, a lot of things began to come clear. To doctors, sickness is a constant presence. They spend their days in a distorted environment, where everyone who comes to see them is sick and in need of help (or at least thinks she is). Try to imagine how your view of life would change if, year after year, you spent every working day dealing with people who are sick, some of them very sick. Would pain and distress begin to seem ordinary? Would you get so used to powerful drugs and invasive operations that they became routine?

When I realized that I was expected to accept both chemotherapy and tamoxifen after my surgery, despite the fact that both have severe side effects and neither was likely to help me, I began to see that chemotherapy, drugs, surgery, and other invasive procedures are commonplace to the doctors who recommend them. When they said they would fix me up with a hysterectomy should tamoxifen cause cancer in my uterus, I realized that to them, the removal of body parts is routine. Treatments I saw as cataclysmic seemed completely ordinary to them.

These are not unfeeling or uncaring people. They are professionals doing what they have been trained to do. They are the carefully molded products of a medical education and a health-care system that have taught them to focus all of their powers and attention on aggressively interceding against disease, and have forgotten to teach them to see the person who carries the disease.

In his thoughtful introduction to Norman Cousins's *The Healing Heart*,[36] Dr. Bernard Lown, a professor at the Harvard University School of Public Health, laments the way technology has crowded communication and personal connection out of medical care, and wonders, "How have physicians grown to be purveyors of biotechnology?" He partly attributes doctors' emphasis on drugs and highly technical treatments to the fact that medical schools select for admission "very bright, achievement-oriented students who have accumulated top grades in scientific subjects" but "often have neglected interpersonal relations." In addition, he says, "the medical-school curriculum dehumanizes even those who come with deeply held aspirations to serve. The four-year, intensive indoctrination aims to instill scientific competence and train bioscientists to manage massive complex technology. Little time or effort is devoted to the cultivation of caring."

Our medical schools create highly skilled technicians and send them out into a field that is perhaps too long on new technologies and drugs, and is certainly too short on time, conversation, and personal connection. It is encouraging that some medical educators, like Dr. Lown, have identified this trend as a problem and are trying to reverse it. In the meantime, there already are, and always have been, doctors who combine their technical skills and knowledge with open communication and genuine caring. They are the ones to look for. There are many others, I believe, who are capable of moving in that direction—and will, if they are pushed to do so by patients who speak up, ask questions, and are willing to share the responsibility for their health care.

Feisty Patients Get More from the System

If you like your doctor but he seems to be too caught up in statistics and technology, remind him that you are an individual and you want to be sure whatever treatments you get fit your body and your lifestyle. That's not being a difficult patient; it's holding up your end of the medical partnership. Your doctor, on the other hand, should be keeping you focused on your medical concerns, and should speak up if you seem to be getting sidetracked by nonhealth issues. Unfortunately, in the case of breast cancer, it is often the doctor who strays into the areas of fashion, psychology, and cosmetic surgery, where he is no expert and doesn't belong. You may be the one who has to bring your doctor back to concentrating on your health.

You may also have to curb your doctor's tendency to prescribe drugs too quickly or needlessly. Overmedication is a real concern in American health care; it masks some problems, creates others, and generally feeds a national drug dependency of mammoth proportions. This, rather than street drugs, is America's major drug problem.

Remember that most doctors today, especially those in urban areas, are overburdened and working under extremely stressful conditions. They are caught between wanting to serve their patients better, which would mean giving each patient more time, and having to follow the rules of increasingly powerful HMOs and insurance companies, which are constantly pressuring them to do more in less time. I don't think doctors like the direction in which medical practice is moving any more than their patients do.

You, as a patient, have more power than you think to ensure that you get the attention you need. At my HMO, I usually can feel that my doctors, even while they are talking to me, are anxious to move on to the next patient. And yet, every time I have spoken up and said I needed to talk a bit more, they have stopped, listened, and responded.

Realize that your doctor has other patients waiting, probably too many. Don't be greedy, but if you still have questions and misgivings, if you need a few minutes more, ask for them. You are no more important to your doctor than the patient waiting to see him next, but you are no less important either. In the long run, one of the most important things your doctor can do for you is to help build a relationship within which you feel comfortable confiding your needs and fears. The two of you need to understand each other. You're going to have to make some big decisions together.

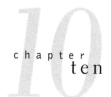
Think Before
You Choose
Your Treatment

*Nobody really
knows much about
breast cancer.*

I hadn't followed breast cancer news stories all that closely before I found my own breast lumps, but I was aware that breast cancer and breast cancer research had moved into the national spotlight, and I believed that medical science was making significant progress. I told myself I was going to have things a lot easier than my mother did facing her breast cancer nearly 30 years ago. That expectation made it all the more amazing and disconcerting to me to discover how little is really known about breast cancer....

As I moved through the many stages of diagnostic testing and treatment, I was struck by the inconclusiveness of every test short of surgical biopsy, and the uncertainty that surrounded every treatment I was offered. I slowly came to accept the stunning fact that after all these years, and all the progress made with other diseases, breast cancer is still essentially an unsolved mystery. Nobody knows what causes it to occur in one woman rather than another, or how to prevent it, or what treatments or lifestyle changes will stop it, or whether it is likely to recur after all signs of it have been successfully obliterated. The enormity of medical ignorance about breast cancer guarantees that every woman who develops the disease is an unwitting player in one of the world's biggest high-stakes games of chance.

How well you do in the first round of the breast cancer game depends, first, on how early you find your tumor, and second, on how careful your doctor is about checking it out. My doctors doggedly sent me from test to test, although they were fairly certain my lumps were not cancer. I sometimes wonder what I would have done if they had simply reassured me and sent me home. Would I have pursued more testing on my own, or, not knowing any better, heaved a sigh of relief and ignored the lumps while they continued to grow and perhaps sent out malignant cells to colonize other parts of my body? I honestly don't know. But you learn very quickly in the breast cancer game that ignorance is not bliss; it is dangerous, and can be fatal. If you want to have any chance at all of winning, you need to know what cards you are holding.

No Easy Answers

❋

I wish I could say that once cancer is detected and conclusively identified, medical knowledge replaces ignorance. Unfortunately, that is not the case. When you learn that you have breast cancer, one doubt is eliminated, but it is quickly replaced by many more. You have breast cancer. You need to treat it. What do you do? A variety of treatments exist, but none is certain to cure, and each presents its own dangers.

Unless your tumor is extremely small, you will have to make decisions about both initial and follow-up treatments. The purpose of the initial treatment is to remove the tumor that already exists. The follow-up treatment attempts to keep the cancer from coming back and from spreading to other parts of your body. In most instances, the first treatment is surgery, but not always. Doctors sometimes recommend radiation or chemotherapy before surgery, to shrink a large tumor to a more manageable size. The surgery itself can be either a mastectomy or a lumpectomy. Lumpectomy almost always means radiation as well. After surgery, possible follow-up treatments usually include radiation, chemotherapy, and the drug tamoxifen.

If it were possible to know how extensive the cancer in your breast is, whether it has already begun to spread beyond the breast, and how aggressive it is going to be, then the choice of treatment would be easier. As it is, before treatment begins, nobody knows. Doctors look at your tests, measure what they see against existing medical statistics and their own experience, and make their best guess as to what to recommend. That's all any of us can expect right now and in the foreseeable future. Breast cancer treatment is largely a judgment call, which is why if you consult three different doctors, you are likely to get three different recommendations. In the end, you are the one who has to choose. Any woman who's been there can tell you it is horribly frustrating. It is infuriating to have to make such a major decision with so little information, but that is the situation we are all in.

The best, most honest doctors admit that they, too, are working mostly in the dark. They, like you, are trying to make the best possible decisions based on what little they know.

To put the situation bluntly, every breast cancer treatment is a gamble. This is a fact that takes some getting used to. We Americans like to believe there is an answer to every problem. Years of drug company advertising have convinced us that regardless of how we abuse our bodies—poor diet, insufficient exercise, rampant pollution, high levels of stress—when we get sick there will be some pill we can pop to set us right. Well, there is no magic pill, or surgery, or radiation treatment for breast cancer. There are only therapies that help some patients and fail others.

Since you, the patient, will ultimately have to choose your treatment, it is important to understand something about how your doctor will arrive at his recommendation. Doctors are painfully aware that any therapy they recommend may or may not help. Having little solid knowledge about your particular cancer and what it is likely to do, they depend heavily on statistics and generalizations. In this way, your doctor's thinking is very different from yours.

A patient's concern is completely egocentric, as it should be. You are worried about your health and your life. You expect your doctor to see you as a unique person with very specific needs. But he can't. Not knowing you or your body, he can't see what is causing your problem. Personally, he may care very much about you as an individual, but medically, he sees you as part of a group that consists of all the women who are known to have suffered the same symptoms that you are describing. He knows from the medical literature what treatments have been tried in similar cases and what percentage of patients have benefited. He bases his recommendation on those statistics.

Doctors also know that a certain percentage of women who have undergone any given treatment have suffered unpleasant and perhaps serious side effects. There are always side effects. In the medical world, a treatment that has benefited a majority of patients and has caused few serious side effects is considered a positive, dependable treatment. Your doctor understands that there is no such thing as a perfect treatment that benefits everyone and hurts no one. You may not ever have thought about that—I hadn't, until I had to decide which breast cancer treatments I would agree to.

Weighing the Alternatives

The concept of justifiable risks and acceptable side effects was new to me, but it is a basic premise that underlies just about everything doctors do. To them, a small percentage of extreme adverse effects is acceptable, if a drug or other treatment is generally effective. As a patient, you need to weigh any risk carefully. The risk may be as low as 1 percent, but if you turn out to be the one patient in a hundred that suffers a serious side effect, for you the impact will be 100 percent. The potential side effects of powerful drugs and surgery range from mild to severe, and sometimes include death.

I am saying this not to frighten you, but rather to impress on you the importance of finding out all you can about any treatment your doctor proposes. Ask what its rate of success has been in cases similar to yours. Ask about possible side effects and how often they occur. You may find, as I did, that your idea of an acceptable risk differs from your doctor's.

You also need to know that the official measure of success for a treatment is often not a cure but simply survival. The medical record-keepers evaluate treatments by counting how many patients are still alive five or ten or more years down the road. The statistics do not describe what those lives are like. A woman who regains her health and resumes her full and happy life shows up in the statistics as a survivor. So does the woman who is suffering from severe side effects or whose cancer has returned and is spreading painfully through her body. To you and me, those women are in completely different worlds; to the statisticians, they are indistinguishable.

Although doctors will cite survival rates, most are reluctant to declare any breast cancer patient cured, for fear the disease may reappear some time in the future and prove them wrong. Nevertheless, many, many women, including myself and my mother, have resumed a normal, healthy life after a bout of breast cancer. There are now millions of former breast cancer patients in the U.S. alone. So when you consider possible treatments, resist the inevitable feelings of urgency and desperation, and choose thoughtfully, as if you're going to live with the results of your choice for a long time. You probably will.

Establish Criteria That Make Sense to You

I don't think it is possible for a layman to understand completely what each breast cancer treatment entails, let alone the subtleties of choosing between one set of chemotherapy drugs and another. We can grasp the basics, though, and put them in a context that makes sense to us.

To find out all you need to know about various treatments, you will have to ask a lot of questions and do some research on your own. You will also need to give serious thought to your own feelings about the quality of your life.

Too many treatment recommendations are based on popular—and, I think, condescending—assumptions about "what women want." This is especially true in choices between mastectomy and lumpectomy and in decisions for or against cosmetic reconstructive surgery, but assumptions are also made as to how much women are willing to suffer for a slightly improved chance of survival. Make sure you know, and that your doctor knows, what's important to you in your life, what you are willing to risk and what you are not. It is important that you feel that whatever treatment you choose is the best one for you. If you believe it gives you the best chance for recovery, your confidence will contribute to its effectiveness. The fear and negativity that come with a treatment you have been pressured into against your better judgment will bring you down, and will work against your healing.

I found that comparing potential treatments became easier when I categorized them according to how extensively and how deeply they would affect my body. I was always optimistic about beating my cancer, so I was concerned not only about how any treatment I chose would affect my tumors, but also about the impact it would have on my overall health once my cancer crisis was over.

I set up three categories. A treatment was either local, meaning it would affect only the breast area; or it was regional, meaning it would also affect the surrounding areas; or it was systemic, meaning it would affect my entire body. It seemed obvious to me that a local treatment posed less of a threat to my postcancer health than a regional one, and both of those were less dangerous than one that was systemic. As I looked at each treatment, I weighed its probable benefits against its potential side effects.

Surgery

I chose to have a mastectomy rather than a lumpectomy because mastectomy is a local treatment, the only breast cancer treatment that is truly local. In a mastectomy, a surgeon removes the entire breast containing the tumor, as well as some or all of the lymph nodes adjoining the breast, through which the cancer may have begun to spread. It's pretty straightforward. The operation itself takes just a few hours, and recovery and healing are rapid. Of course, every treatment has its side effects. The most common problem after mastectomy is stiffness or limited arm mobility. (I didn't have either.) Simple exercise or physical therapy usually helps. Because their lymph nodes are gone, some women (about 10 percent) have problems with fluid collecting in the arm on the surgery side, a condition called lymphedema.[37] It can be quite uncomfortable and, if severe, may require regular draining.

Of course, anesthesia poses a risk with any kind of surgery, but it is a very small one statistically. Other than the anesthesia, mastectomy doesn't invade your body very deeply. Your breast, after all, is external; that is, outside of the area where your vital organs reside. I liked the fact that the outcome of mastectomy is pretty predictable—not as to whether it will successfully stop your cancer (that depends on whether the cancer has already started to spread) but as to what physical impact it will have on your body. In short, you will be left with a flat scar where your breast once was. To me, that's a very minor drawback for a treatment that has a long-established record for effectiveness, especially with early-stage tumors. Lots of healthy, one-breasted women are living happy lives thanks to a timely mastectomy.

I have seen mastectomy referred to as the most severe of the breast cancer treatments, even as barbaric, because it removes the entire breast. To my mind, mastectomy is the most benign of the available treatments, because it is the least invasive and has the fewest potentially harmful side effects.

Many women choose lumpectomy over mastectomy because it removes just the tumor and the tissue surrounding it, leaving the breast pretty much intact. It is true that the results of lumpectomy are cosmetically more pleasing than those of mastectomy. If lumpectomy were as effective as mastectomy in stopping cancer, I would have chosen it. But even its most ardent advocates do not claim that i t is. Because no one believes that lumpectomy will stop breast cancer, it is automatically paired with a powerful second treatment, radiation, which moves it out of the local treatment category into the regional category. Even followed by radiation, lumpectomy is not as effective as mastectomy.

There always seems to be variation in medical statistics, but the numbers I have seen most often comparing lumpectomy and mastectomy assert that 10 percent of women who undergo lumpectomy with radiation have local recurrences of their breast cancer, compared to 8 percent of women with similar cancers who have mastectomies. [38] That means that a woman who chooses lumpectomy over mastectomy increases her chances of a recurrence by 25 percent. Still, many doctors assume that female vanity will push a woman to choose lumpectomy over mastectomy, and, amazingly to me, many feminist activists champion it.

In her book *To Dance with The Devil: The New War on Breast Cancer,* journalist Karen Stabiner suggests that women who have chosen lumpectomy "considered it a political issue—a symbol of liberation from a male-dominated medical establishment they increasingly regarded as being more interested in heroics than in a woman's self-image." [39] Personally, I think a lot of women who choose lumpectomy have been misled by widely published claims that the two procedures produce equal results. To evaluate lumpectomy intelligently, you have

to consider not only the surgery, but the effects of the radiation therapy that comes with it.

Radiation

The radiation used in conjunction with lumpectomy is much more
controlled and focused these days than it once was, but it is still a powerful cell-destroying force that affects more than the immediate breast
area. "In the old days, we used a cobalt machine that was aimed at the
general area instead of a carefully plotted site, and the radiation scat-
tered a lot," Dr. Susan Love says in her best-selling *Dr. Susan Love's
Breast Book*. In trying to radiate the breast, "you also radiat[ed] the
lungs, and, if it's the left breast, the heart." With today's more precise
technology, she says, "the radiation goes through a particular breast
area and out into air, and less into your heart or lung." [40]

As Love describes it, radiation treatments are given five days a week
for five or six weeks, using about 4,700 rads or centigrays of radiation.
For comparison, she offers that a chest x-ray is just a fraction of a rad. I
never seriously considered lumpectomy because the thought of radiation frightened me. As I have read more about it, I am convinced I
made the right decision.

Radiation is used in the treatment of many cancers, and in most
cases it does eradicate the cancer cells remaining in the breast after
lumpectomy, so in the short term it is an effective breast cancer
treatment. The problem is that no one knows for certain what long-
term effects it has on the body. When it comes to my health, I admit
to having a great fear of the unknown. In her book *To Be Alive: A
Woman's Guide to a Full Life After Cancer*, Dr. Carolyn Runowicz,
Director of the Division of Gynecologic Oncology at the Albert
Einstein College of Medicine in New York, worries about what she

calls "a disturbing array of long-term and late effects" from radiation. Where surgery and radiation are used together, she says, some women develop chronic pain because radiation leaves behind scar tissue that can entrap and injure nerves. She cautions that radiation "can weaken the function of certain critical organs like the heart, lungs, and kidneys" and that "the risks of later complications persist for more than 25 years after treatment." [41]

There is also concern among radiation oncologists, including prominent researcher and author O. Carl Simonton, that radiation affects the immune system, weakening it for as long as two years after treatment. [42]

Dr. Susan Love touches on a number of lesser side effects in her book, ranging from a "sunburn" on the skin to nausea, diarrhea, hair loss, coughing, asymptomatic rib fractures, fatigue (which can last for months), and depression. "Your breast will never feel completely normal again," she says; "you'll continue to have some sharp, shooting pains from time to time." As for cosmetic results, the main selling point for lumpectomy with radiation, she warns, "a large amount of radiation will always be somewhat cosmetically displeasing, since it can cause permanent swelling in the breast as well as thickened skin." [43]

Joyce Wadler, who told the story of her own cancer experience in *My Breast: One Woman's Cancer Story*, was warned by her radiation therapist that her irradiated breast could become as much as a cup size larger or smaller as a result of radiation. In addition, most doctors seem to agree, as Wadler's doctor warned her, that "there is a great deal of internal scarring, which can interfere with getting a good picture on a mammogram." [44]

For all these reasons, lumpectomy followed by radiation seemed to me far less desirable than mastectomy. That was my choice. Your choice, after weighing the cosmetic and health advantages of the two surgeries and your own concerns about your appearance, may be the same or different. Choose what is best for you, but don't choose without careful consideration.

Follow-Up Therapy

When you undergo breast surgery, you quickly learn a few critical new phrases. One is "dirty margins." The breast tissue removed by a surgeon is examined by a pathologist under a microscope. If malignant cells reach all the way to the edge, it has dirty margins, which means there are probably still cancer cells in whatever remains of the breast. "If it's on one side of the scalpel, it's probably on the other," as Dr. S. put it. I was lucky. I had clean margins, and no sign of cancer in any of the 45 lymph nodes that were removed. "Your report is an A-plus," he told me. Still, I had to face the question of follow-up therapy, and you probably will too.

If you're among the many women who emerge from surgery as I did with clean lymph nodes and no detectable cancer left in your body, you may think you can just walk away from breast cancer, back to a healthy life. It's not that simple. Dr. S. explained the situation this way: It is the current medical belief that seven out of ten women like us are indeed cured and will never have a recurrence. It's a triumphant statistic, but there's a catch: no one has yet come up with a way of identifying which seven.

Of the three out of ten who will have recurrences, statistics say two will die no matter what treatments they undergo. There's no way of knowing who they are either. The remaining one will have a recurrence but can be helped by chemotherapy, which is a nasty experience by anybody's standards, but worth it if it saves your life.

I don't know how many researchers are trying to find the key to this particular prognosis puzzle. I hope there are many. If there were a test that could identify the three in ten who are actually still in danger, 70 percent of the thousands of women whose cancer is caught before it leaves the breast would be spared the agonizing choice between the horrors of chemotherapy and the frightening uncertainty of turning it down. [45] Perhaps, too, if such a test existed, doctors would be less worried about the threat of malpractice suits, which now pressures them to recommend dangerous follow-up therapies for just about everyone, even when they know how few will be helped.

I declined chemotherapy, feeling that a one-in-ten chance that it might help was not enough to balance the invasiveness of the treatment and the dangers of its side effects. I believe I am in the minority. According to the oncologist I consulted, most women in my position are afraid to take the chance and so choose to have chemo. As a result, every year thousands of healthy women undergo a physically devastating, expensive treatment they don't need, simply because no one has figured out yet how to tell who needs it and who doesn't.

Chemotherapy

While surgery alone is local, and surgery with radiation is regional, chemotherapy is systemic. It affects your entire body. Doctors believe that breast cancer can spread if just one microscopic malignant cell manages to travel to another part of the body and grow there. It can start growing immediately or wait for years. Since there is still no way to know whether or to which body part the cancer has spread, oncologists usually recommend following breast cancer surgery with chemotherapy, which infuses the patient's body with highly toxic chemicals that kill any fast-growing cells they come into contact with. Cancer cells, which are usually fast-growing, are the primary target, but other fast-growing cells, such as hair cells, are destroyed too. The side effects of chemotherapy range from the uncomfortable—nausea, hair loss, and fatigue—to the extremely dangerous—damage to vital organs, development of new cancers, and suppression of the immune system.

The latter effect particularly frightened me. The oncologist who recommended I have chemo said I would have to be extremely wary of infections if I underwent treatment. Any infection could become serious, possibly even fatal, because my immune system would be too weak to counteract it. He didn't mention the fact that I had an 8-year-old daughter at the time, or that kids are always bringing home colds and other infections. It didn't occur to me, either, in the midst of all the other risks I was trying to evaluate, until a friend mentioned that a woman she knew was advised not to see her grandchildren during her months of chemotherapy. She also told me about a young public defender who had to stay away from work because of all the people bringing colds and other infections into his busy office. Given my family situation, I couldn't imagine how I could protect myself. I decided I would be crazy to knock out my immune system at a time in my life when I really needed it. Chemotherapy as a possible cure for an existing cancer might still have made sense to me; for a precautionary measure, with only a 10 percent chance of helping, the risk seemed too high.

Some doctors have concluded that damage to the immune system is also the reason chemotherapy sometimes leads to new cancers. Dr. Deepak Chopra, best-selling author and popular lecturer on health, thinks the danger is especially high for breast cancer patients. In his 1989 book *Quantum Healing* he says that many chemotherapy drugs "directly suppress the bone marrow, which manufactures our white blood cells, with devastating effect on the white-cell count in the blood. As the course of therapy continues, the patient becomes more and more susceptible to new forms of cancer, and in a certain number of cases—as high as 30 percent for breast cancer—new cancer appears and the patient dies." [46]

As I accumulated my information on chemotherapy, one of the biggest surprises to me was that it is not as effective as I had always assumed. Most sources, including Dr. Susan Love, peg chemotherapy as about 33 percent effective in stopping the spread of breast cancer and preventing recurrences. *The New Our Bodies, Ourselves,* one of the few health information books that comes from the patient's rather than the medical professional's point of view, is not even that optimistic. It estimates that "chemotherapy in premenopausal women (whether lymph nodes are positive or negative) will reduce mortality from breast cancer by 25 percent." In older women, the authors doubt that it is very effective at all: "Women over 60 have fared as well without chemotherapy as with it." [47]

There are no certainties with breast cancer. If you have metastatic cancer—cancer that has already spread beyond the breast—even a 25 to 33 percent chance of stopping it is probably worth trying for. If you have no remaining signs of cancer after surgery and chemotherapy is offered as a hedge against a possible future recurrence, the choice is not so clear. The doctors I spoke to told me with great certainty that "women want" to have any treatment that might help, despite the dangers and the odds. I think it is a terribly personal decision, and that each woman has to weigh the plusses and minuses of her unique situation. As for "what women want," I think I am safe in projecting that women want someone to come up with a test that identifies which cancers are likely to metastasize and which are not. Beyond that, women want an effective, nonpoisonous treatment for metastatic breast cancer. What women don't want is to keep finding themselves trapped by medical ignorance between the proverbial devil and the deep blue sea.

Tamoxifen

❁

The oncologist who recommended that I undergo chemotherapy to diminish the chances of a breast cancer recurrence recommended that I take tamoxifen for the same purpose, every day, for at least five years. As scary as the thought of chemotherapy was to me, tamoxifen was scarier. Doctors at least have an idea of what chemotherapy drugs are likely to do in your body. Nobody seems to understand what tamoxifen does. That hasn't stopped it from becoming one of the most widely prescribed drugs in the world.

Tamoxifen has been around for about 20 years. Researchers have concluded that it functions a lot like estrogen in a woman's breast, attaching itself to estrogen receptors in potentially cancerous breast tissue. Unlike estrogen, which is thought to spur the growth of cancer, tamoxifen appears to occupy receptor sites without stimulating cancer growth. It therefore reduces the chance of a breast cancer recurrence. Sounds great. Unfortunately, tamoxifen acts differently in other parts of a woman's body. In the uterus, for instance, instead of preventing cancer, it sometimes causes it.

For women who already have metastatic breast cancer, tamoxifen, like chemotherapy, may be worth trying, although it appears to be even less effective than chemo. There is, as always, disagreement among the experts. *The New Our Bodies, Ourselves* estimates that in postmenopausal women, hormone (tamoxifen) therapy reduces mortality by 15 percent.[48] The authors doubt the drug's effectiveness in premenopausal women, however. Journalist Roberta Altman bolsters that doubt, reporting in *Waking Up, Fighting Back* that in a National Surgical Adjuvant Breast and Bowel Project trial, which compared the effectiveness of chemotherapy and tamoxifen in 1900 women with breast cancer, women who were "under the age of 50, or premenopausal, did not benefit from the tamoxifen." [49] In *To Dance with the Devil*, Karen Stabiner quotes a more optimistic Dr. Susan Love telling student doctors that tamoxifen decreases mortality in premenopausal patients by 12 percent and in older women by 29 percent. [50] In *Tamoxifen and Breast Cancer*, authors Michael W. DeGregorio and Valerie J. Wiebe report that in an early study about one-third of postmenopausal women with metastatic breast cancer responded to tamoxifen treatment, and that when both tamoxifen and chemotherapy were used, the response rate went up. They also state, however, that "virtually all patients will eventually develop tamoxifen resistance and no longer respond....[A]fter six months to a year of therapy, the tumor will begin to recur." [51]

As a premenopausal breast cancer patient without any signs of metastatic disease, I found little to encourage me to take tamoxifen as a way of preventing recurrences. The oncologist I consulted explained that while chemotherapy had a one-in-ten chance of doing me some good, tamoxifen had only a 1-in-20 chance. He looked me straight in the eye and said, "We treat the nineteen women who won't be helped for the sake of the twentieth who will." Nineteen women exposed to a daunting range of known and still-to-be-documented side effects, for the sake of one who may benefit for six months or a year?

I searched for information and read that not only does tamoxifen put women at risk for potentially fatal uterine cancer, it has also caused fatal blood clots and is suspected of causing deaths from hepatitis and liver failure, and of contributing to the development of stomach, liver, and colon cancers. [52] Still, doctors who consider the relatively small number of these extreme "side effects" an acceptable risk recommend tamoxifen to women like me as protection.

I felt trapped between the pressure I felt from my doctors to take tamoxifen and my own fears that by doing so I would be poisoning my body. I kept imagining what it would feel like day after day standing in the bathroom, pill in hand, looking at myself in the mirror, terrified. I knew I couldn't do it, but I was afraid to make such a major decision on instinct alone. I made appointments to talk to both my gynecologist and a psychologist at my HMO. The gynecologist told me that she and other doctors in her department had been seeing unexplainable vaginal bleeding in women who were on tamoxifen. The psychologist agreed with me that my fear of the drug could cause psychological and emotional problems, whether or not that fear was justified. That was enough corroboration for me. I refused to take tamoxifen.

Making the Tough Decisions

The hardest part of deciding on a treatment is realizing that there are no sure answers when it comes to breast cancer. The more you read, the more you uncover contradictions. The more doctors you talk to, the more conflicting opinions you hear, and the more you realize that each doctor is convinced that his own approach is the most effective. Medical specialization is in one way a blessing, because it allows a doctor in a demanding field such as surgery or oncology to concentrate on a small, clearly defined area and to become truly expert in it. In another way, specialization is a curse, because it narrows that doctor's focus. Many doctors end up being spokesmen for their fields rather than objective advocates for their patients.

When you consult a specialist, you should assume going in that he chose his particular area of medicine in the first place because it made sense to him, and he's stayed in it because he believes it works. Expect a surgeon to recommend surgery, a radiology oncologist to recommend radiation, a medical oncologist to recommend chemotherapy. But don't assume that all the doctors in the same field see things the same way. Given the lack of knowledge about breast cancer, everyone is guessing.

In *Cancer in Two Voices,* Barbara Rosenblum comments on her desperate visits to several cancer specialists. "Surgeons tend to see breast cancer as a local disease, so they want to cut first. Oncologists see cancer systemically, as an immune system disease, and they say attack with chemotherapy. Then, when I went to see three different oncologists, I got three different opinions anyhow; it threw me into a crisis of uncertainty." [53]

Confusion and uncertainty are the hallmarks of the breast cancer patient. And yet we must choose among the available treatments, and hope we are choosing right. Some women simply let their doctors decide. Once I realized how little the experts actually know, and how their own prejudices and loyalties influence their recommendations, I didn't feel comfortable doing that.

I learned through my own experience how hard it is to reject a doctor's recommendation, but I also learned, to my surprise, that my doctors were ready to accept whatever decision I made, so long as I made it thoughtfully. I have heard stories from other women about doctors refusing to care for a patient who rejects a suggested treatment. That did not happen to me. I think I would have mightily resented any doctor who showed me such disrespect.

If you decide, as I did, to make your own choices, you will probably feel uneasy about your lack of knowledge, but at least you will know that the person doing the choosing is the one who cares most about every aspect of your health. When you evaluate proposed treatments, just take your time, consider all the possibilities, and remember to factor in your own values, instincts, and plans for your future after cancer.

chapter eleven

Be Adventurous

(There'll Never Be
a Better Time)

*Try anything that
might help.*

If you don't know much about so-called alternative therapies, now would be a good time to start learning. Searching for relief from discomfort and anxiety, millions of Americans, including many breast cancer patients, supplement their conventional medical care with alternative treatments. A growing number of doctors are opening their minds to healing methods outside their medical training as well, although they are rightly cautious about recommending approaches about which they have little information....

Let me start with a word of caution. Like all unexplored territories, the world of alternative medicine poses some hidden dangers. There are a lot of well-established treatments and activities available that, while out of the mainstream, have proved successful for many people for a long time. There are also some treatments that sound pretty dubious to me, and some practitioners who sound like quacks. As you start exploring, be open to new ideas, but don't be foolhardy. Read, ask questions, talk to other cancer patients who have tried a treatment that appeals to you. Most of all, pay attention to your own body and emotions, and seek out what makes you feel better and what makes sense to you.

Start right away. Just embarking on the search is a positive step. If the idea of seeking help outside of conventional medical treatments seems frightening, or even disloyal, start with something very simple, like having a massage to help you relax. Once you see how much better it makes you feel, you may be inspired to look for other "nontraditional" ways of dealing with your illness.

I suspect the word "nontraditional" is itself intimidating to some people. It is used a lot these days to stigmatize any treatment that falls outside the current medical mainstream. The fact is, however, that many of the techniques we label nontraditional have been practiced effectively throughout the world for centuries. From a historical perspective, it is our own approach to medicine, so focused on drugs and surgery, that is new, harsh, and nontraditional. Caught up in our love affair with technology, we have lost touch with a whole range of simple, natural healing techniques.

Unexpected Relief

My own first venture into alternative therapies was prompted not by my cancer, but by menopause.[54] In my case, it started a good two years before I discovered my breast tumors. For many women, menopause is a side effect of breast cancer treatment, adding such miseries as hot flashes, irritability, headaches, and insomnia to an already disturbing collection of discomforts.

My first clear symptom was hot flashes. Then came occasional headaches. I had only the vaguest idea of what was happening inside my body until the day I stumbled onto a radio interview with therapist Lonnie Barbach, who was promoting her book *The Pause*.[55] Barbach's positive attitude toward menopause appealed to me. I bought the book and read it from cover to cover. Many of the women Barbach quoted swore by one nonmedical therapy or another, but none seemed particularly pertinent to me at the time.

Some months later, on a stifling summer day, I was leveled by a pounding headache. I took several doses of an over-the-counter painkiller, but it couldn't touch this monster headache, and as the day wore on I grew desperate. Suddenly a paragraph from Barbach's book popped into my mind. One woman had said she learned from an American Indian to rub peppermint oil on her forehead to stop headaches. It didn't seem like it could possibly work, but I was in agony, nothing was helping, and there was a health food store just a few blocks from my house. I convinced my husband to walk over with me.

As I grabbed a bottle of peppermint oil from the shelf, a row of little boxes caught my eye. They contained homeopathic remedies. A purple box in the middle of the display was labeled "menopause." I picked it up and read the back. The name Dana Ullman touched off memories.[56] Ullman is a well-known homeopath from whom I had taken an adult-education class some twenty years earlier. I remembered him as extremely bright and dedicated. His stories of patients he had helped had impressed me as sensible and insightful, but I was just dabbling at the time and had never considered turning to homeopathy for my own health care. Now I thought if Ullman formulated these remedies, they were probably worth trying. They might help, I reasoned, and they couldn't hurt. I've never heard anyone accuse homeopathic remedies of causing negative side effects. I walked out of the store with a bottle of peppermint oil and a box of remedies. The two together cost less than fifteen dollars.

At home I rubbed a little peppermint oil on my forehead, above the bridge of my nose, and immediately cringed at the burning sensation it caused in my eyes. Within a half hour, the worst headache I had ever had was gone. I was amazed. I have used peppermint oil for headaches many times since, as has my husband. Usually it works. Sometimes it doesn't. I don't know why.

The next time I was hit with a hot flash, out came the homeopathic remedies. I placed one of the little white tablets under my tongue and waited while it slowly dissolved. My body temperature returned to normal so quickly I was sure it couldn't have had anything to do with the remedy. Next hot flash, another tablet, with the same result. "Once an accident, twice a coincidence," the saying goes. But three times, that's a pattern. The third time the result was the same, and I was sold. I was soon using the remedies for my other menopausal symptoms, both physical (insomnia) and emotional (irritability), with equally positive results.

There was one failure. After about a year of success in fighting middle-of-the-night insomnia, the menopause remedies stopped helping. I tried switching to the formula specifically for insomnia, and that continues to work. My whole family now uses homeopathic remedies for cold and flu symptoms, and my husband uses them to relieve minor injuries he brings home from the soccer field.

I don't understand why either the peppermint oil or the remedies work. I've read medical researchers' arguments that homeopathic remedies can't possibly be effective because the active ingredients are diluted so many times there isn't enough left to supply even a single molecule for each little tablet. Frankly, I don't care if they don't make sense to scientists. I only care that they help me.

Do We Have Too Much Science?

It's not that I don't respect science. I do. Scientists have untangled a lot of mysteries and solved a lot of problems, but the fact that they cannot measure or prove something doesn't mean it doesn't exist or doesn't work. There are many, many things that scientists can't explain. I think as a society we have blinded ourselves to the shortcomings of science and are afraid to point out its negative impacts. Thanks to the wonders of modern technology, an alarming number of us live mostly sedentary lives, eat packaged foods at home and fast food everywhere else, live surrounded by polluted air and water, and work in buildings where the light is artificial and the windows are sealed shut. Over the last half-century, we have been lulled into a feeling of well-being by a never-ending parade of new products, while we have become increasingly susceptible to diseases like breast cancer.

Fifty years ago, an American woman's lifetime risk of getting breast cancer was estimated at one in twenty. Today it is estimated at one in eight. You can argue with the exact numbers, and I am one who does, but you can't escape the fact that a lot more women are getting breast cancer today than in our grandmothers' time. Obviously, we're doing something wrong.

I think one of the biggest mistakes we've made is turning health care into sick care, and making it the exclusive province of experts and professionals. Once you accept the idea that health care is scientific, it seems very complicated, and it's hard to believe you know how to take care of yourself. When it comes to caring for our bodies, most of us ignore our common sense and depend instead on the dictates of others. We don't think seriously about our health until it fails us. When we do get sick, we don't say, "Maybe I'm pushing myself too hard" or "I've got to start eating more vegetables." We go to a doctor, and usually come out with a drug prescription. Our lifestyle stays the same, but we think we're taking care of ourselves because we're taking drugs.

I was interviewed by a lot of medical people during my cancer testing and treatment, and every one of them went through a long checklist of drugs I might be taking. I told them I wasn't taking any drugs, but they kept reading off the list. They seemed certain that a woman my age must be taking something. I began to realize that most American women my age do take drugs regularly, and they're not the only ones. A major portion of our population has become drug-dependent.

Many of us have accepted the idea that drugs are a reasonable substitute for a healthful lifestyle. We have let ourselves be convinced that it is not only possible but perfectly sensible to fill our nutritional needs by popping pills rather than eating well. The practice has become so commonplace, especially among "health-conscious" people, we hardly think to question it. These days as soon as a food is demonstrated to be important to good health, someone sets out to isolate its essential nutrient and turn it into a pill—and millions of Americans start popping. We've been seduced by one alphabet vitamin after another, by beta carotene, by folic acid. The fact that these isolated nutrients don't benefit the body in the same way they do in their natural state somehow gets lost in the excitement. In fact, when a beta carotene pill was tried out as a protection against lung cancer, it didn't decrease the number of deaths, it increased them. [57] Still, we would rather take pills than eat well, and science continues to push us in that direction.

Personally, I think it's time to tell the researchers we're tired of being put on pills. And it's time to admit to ourselves that we know how to stay healthy. We've just been too lazy to do much about it. I've learned from my own experience that once you begin taking responsibility for your own health on a very basic level—improving your diet and exercising more, for instance—your attitude toward your body changes, and you begin looking at all your health-care choices with new confidence in your own judgment.

Put Yourself in Charge
of Your Well-Being

Don't think that if you've already got cancer it's too late to start changing your unhealthy habits. You may be sick, but you intend to survive, and you'll be better off with healthier habits in the future. The easiest, most obvious way for most people to start is to improve their diet. The average American diet is a disaster—too high in fat, sugar, and salt, and too low in fruits, vegetables, nuts, and grains. Although the link between diet and health seems obvious to an ordinary person like me, the experts, as usual, can't agree. The argument is especially vigorous on the question of whether diet has an impact on breast cancer.

On one side is the eat-less-fat contingent. A 1991 article in *Time* magazine observed, "The United States, Great Britain, and the Netherlands, countries in which the consumption of fat is high, have among the highest breast cancer rates, whereas in Japan, Singapore, and Rumania, where a very lean diet is eaten, the incidence of breast cancer is one-sixth to one-half the rate in the United States." [58] It may be hard to prove a cause-and-effect connection, but the statistics are pretty convincing in themselves, and pretty frightening. In her book *Waking Up, Fighting Back*, Roberta Altman reports that a study published in 1995 found that women in Greece who were cancer-free consumed more fruits, vegetables, and olive oil than those who developed breast cancer. [59] Altman also cites a 1991 article in the *Journal of the National Cancer Institute* that contains actual numbers, estimating that every 693 calories of fat consumed in a day increases a woman's risk of breast cancer by 35 percent. [60]

Those on the diet-doesn't-matter side of the argument most often cite a widely publicized study of American nurses, whose breast cancer rate turned out to be the same regardless of what they ate. [61] The oncologist I consulted referred to this study as if it were the last word on the subject. Unfortunately, the nurses involved, being American, had diets that ranged from 27 to 50 percent fat. Even those at the low end were eating a high-fat diet by most countries' standards. The Japanese diet, for instance, is closer to 10 to 15 percent fat.

In February 1996 the *New York Times* reported that "a prestigious scientific panel" had concluded that "about one-third of the nation's 1.35 million new cancer cases each year could be traced to diet." [62] They recommended that Americans eat fewer calories, fewer fats, and more fruits and vegetables.

Little Changes Add Up

Eating well isn't as difficult as you might think. I'm neither a fanatic nor an expert on the subject, but I've made it my business to know the basic concepts of healthful eating. With a little research and a little thought, you can pinpoint your bad eating habits and begin to change them. I have my own personal smart-eating guidelines, which are pretty simple: Avoid most processed foods, especially those that contain fake anything, and fried foods. Eat lots of fresh fruits and vegetables. And try for as much variety as possible. That's it. I discovered, to my delight, that I already like eating many of the foods researchers say protect you from cancer, including broccoli, tofu, and garlic, so I eat them frequently. But in general, if you eat real (as opposed to manufactured) food that's fresh, in season, and abundant, you can't go far wrong.

To find out what's in season, all you have to do is visit the produce section of your supermarket. Here are two good pieces of advice I've recently heard. The first came from a food-writer friend, who tells her readers to shop the perimeter of the supermarket, where most of the fresh food is, and avoid the middle, which is full of packaged, processed things. The second came from a surgeon I heard speak at a breast cancer seminar. She said her grandmother, now in her nineties, always told her to "eat colors." Colorful foods—those that are naturally green, orange, yellow, red—are usually high in vitamins and other important nutrients. To those tips I would add: read labels. The nutrition information you need is right there on most packages.

I already had pretty good eating habits, being married to a food writer, but after my mastectomy I decided to cut all the fat I could from my diet. It surprised me how easy it was to make changes. I was in the habit of munching on peanuts in that hour before dinner when I was too hungry to wait. Peanuts are about 70 percent fat. I switched to pretzels that have no fat, and painlessly eliminated my worst eating habit.

My next target was ice cream, which I love. I switched to sorbet. It has no fat and wasn't much of a sacrifice. I still eat ice cream occasionally, and chocolate cake too. I'm not going to totally give up foods I like, because I don't want to live that way. I don't think doctors who tell cancer patients to adhere to a strict diet take into consideration the stress that comes with dieting. The constant struggle to control your desires has got to be harder on your body than an occasional candy bar. We Americans seem to have a hard time with the concept of moderation. If too much of something is bad, we assume we shouldn't have any at all. Especially when it comes to food and drink, we're always on a seesaw. Strict denial leads to a frenzy of overindulgence, which sends us guiltily back to denial. Unless you're a fast-food addict, I don't believe you have to completely overhaul your eating habits to improve your health. Every step in the right direction helps. The next time you start to reach for a bag of potato chips, eat a piece of fresh fruit instead, and you'll be on your way.

Exercise, of course, is as important to good health as diet. Even the experts agree on this one, although they argue about how much exercise and what kind we need. A 14-year study of more than 25,000 Norwegian women, published in the *New England Journal of Medicine* in 1997, found that those who exercised regularly had a 37 percent lower incidence of breast cancer. Those who did heavy manual labor at work had a 52 percent lower risk. [63] Those risk-lowering rates are better than any I've seen for drugs, and all the side effects are beneficial. The study defined exercise as four or more hours a week of physical exercise strenuous enough to raise the woman's heart rate and cause her to sweat.

I was once an avid racquetball player, and for a while I jogged every morning before work, but I stopped exercising regularly when my daughter was born in 1986. After I healed from my breast surgery, my husband and I decided to join the YMCA and start playing racquetball again. We went for a tour of the Oakland Y, which turned out to be way too expensive. In fact, all the formal exercise options we looked into — classes, membership clubs — were beyond our budget. I began to think I couldn't afford to exercise, which was a depressing thought. Once I got over my initial frustration, I realized there are still some things you can do for free. Like walk. Now I save trips to the bank, post office, and grocery store for lunchtime and do them on foot, which means I walk for at least half an hour every workday. On weekends we do longer family hikes or go for bicycle rides.

My daughter loves soccer, and sometimes we take the ball to a park near our house and kick it around. In addition to getting my own exercise and having a lot of fun, I like to think I'm encouraging her to stay active. Dr. Susan Love has been quoted as telling a women's luncheon audience, "The biggest thing we can do to prevent osteoporosis, heart disease, and breast cancer is to promote grammar school and high school athletics for girls." [64]

It's encouraging that some doctors are beginning to separate themselves from the heavily drug-focused medical mainstream and say what should be obvious to us all: if you pay attention to your body's basic needs for good food, exercise, and relaxation, you can greatly reduce your need for medical intervention. Perhaps one day we'll all realize that living well is not only the best revenge, it is also the best protection, and the cheapest form of health care.

While we're talking about bad habits, it needs to be said that smoking increases breast cancer risk. A recent study, done in Switzerland, showed that both active and passive exposure to tobacco smoke can triple a woman's risk of getting breast cancer. [65] The American Cancer Society says that if you are a smoker you not only increase your risk of getting the disease, you increase your risk of dying from it, by 25 percent if you smoke at all and by as much as 75 percent if you smoke two or more packs a day. [66] If the threat of breast cancer isn't enough, the

National Cancer Institute adds that the risk of death from all smoking-related diseases has more than doubled since the 1950s and has risen fastest among women. [67]

A Gentler Approach

❋

Improving your daily habits will make you healthier, but that alone will not cure your breast cancer. Nor will alternative therapies replace current mainstream treatments any time soon. Some alternative therapies, however, do offer benign ways of dealing with the unpleasant side effects of mainstream treatments, including stress and other psychological problems.

I have tried only a few alternative methods, so I can speak from experience only about them. Of those I have not tried, I know many have been extremely helpful to others. A friend who has recovered from advanced ovarian cancer swears by Chinese herbs. I have talked to many women who have found relief, from both stress and physical symptoms, in massage, acupuncture and acupressure, and meditation. Whenever I hear their stories, I am struck by how well these different approaches work—and by how many of us continue to be amazed that they do. Perhaps it is time to simply accept that there are many paths to relief, both physical and mental, and to be bold in seeking out the particular treatments that suit us.

I was doubtful, as I have said, about the abilities of peppermint oil to relieve my headaches and homeopathic remedies to control my menopausal symptoms. That doubt was mild, however, compared to my early skepticism about visualization, one of the mind-body therapies that has begun to spread from New Age enclaves to the fringes of mainstream medicine. Back in the early 1980s I was a freelancer hired to edit several New Age channeled books. The two authors I worked closely with were always talking about using visualization to create things they wanted—everything from a parking space in a crowded neighborhood to some physical change in their bodies. I would usually smile noncommittally and steer the conversation onto another subject.

Then one day my husband was chopping kale with a big French knife and sliced off the tip of a finger. I ran into the kitchen to find him pale and bleeding, his fingertip lying on the cutting board. I picked it up and helped him set it back in place. We wrapped a damp paper towel around the finger and made a beeline for the emergency room. The surgeon on duty was not encouraging. He said sometimes with children a piece of flesh like that would reattach, but never with adults. He said he'd sew the fingertip back on if that's what we wanted, but it would just turn black and fall off. We wanted to try, so he painstakingly stitched the little piece of tissue in place, bandaged it, and sent us on our way.

At home I found myself urging Jay to use visualization to try to get his fingertip to reattach. I couldn't believe I was doing it, and I couldn't believe he agreed. I guess we both felt there was nothing to lose. Every day he would sit for about fifteen minutes with his eyes closed, picturing the little piece of flesh reattaching itself to his finger. Two weeks went by, and he returned to the hospital to have the bandage removed. To his amazement, only the top layer of skin had turned black; underneath, the tissue was pink and healthy, and firmly attached. Today the finger looks completely normal; you can barely see the scar.

My own first attempt at visualization came a dozen years later, the week before my mastectomy. We were on vacation in Hawaii, and during the day I hardly thought about my upcoming surgery, but in bed at night I worried that my cancer might have already spread. I decided to try using my mind to get any escaped cancer cells to move back into the breast so that they'd be removed with it. Every night, after Jay dropped off to sleep, I lay quietly beside him picturing the maverick cells being drawn from various parts of my body back into my left breast. I actually felt tingling in my limbs as I visualized the process, until the last night, when I didn't feel anything at all. I told myself the job must be done, but I can't say I really believed any of it. A few days later my breast was surgically removed, and with it all detectable signs of cancer. Did my visualization exercises contribute to that result? I'll never know.

Despite those two experiences, I wasn't really convinced of the powers of visualization until recently, when I performed my own little lab test. One day, out of nowhere, a mole appeared on my back. I didn't think it was dangerous in any way, but I hated it being there, and it was soon surrounded by a scaly patch of psoriasis, my body's way of marking areas of stress (as if I need to have them pointed out). I decided to see if I could make the whole offensive mess disappear by visualizing its destruction.

Each morning after my shower I stood naked for about 30 seconds, rubbing a psoriasis ointment on the spot and imagining my body drawing the mole into it, dissolving it bit by bit, and flushing the remnants away. Since I could barely see that part of my back, every few days I asked Jay to check it out. His first progress report was that the mole looked pretty much the same, maybe a tiny bit smaller. He wasn't about to believe that my efforts would succeed. After about a week, however, he was sure the mole was shrinking and the psoriasis pretty much gone. A week after that he found just the tiniest raised spot on my skin. And a few days later, nothing at all. Don't ask me why or how it worked. All I know is that I no longer have a mole on my back and I now believe our bodies have powers to change themselves that we will never explain.

There are many therapies besides visualization that are based on the belief in a powerful mind-body connection. Some start with the mind—meditation, biofeedback, psychotherapy; some start with the body—yoga, tai chi, massage. All have their advocates, and I am certain all of them are helpful in promoting healing, vitality, and ongoing good health. If one or more feel right to you, give them a try. Don't worry if you are the first in your family or among your friends to look outside of standard medical procedures for relief. Be the adventurer, and reap the rewards.

While you're doing all you can for your body, remember the simple things that lift your spirits. Maybe it's being with friends, or working on an art project, or writing poetry, or riding a bicycle, or listening to music. You probably don't think of those things as therapies, but if they improve your mood and brighten your outlook, they qualify in my book. Some scientists are actually starting to believe that such activities provide real physical advantages in addition to the psychological ones we've all experienced. I recently heard of a study that showed listening to music can stimulate the release of endorphins, those natural pain killers our brains supply at no charge and with no side effects. If you listen to music to relax and improve your mood, you're already using an alternative therapy. You're on the cutting edge.

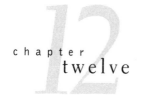

Expect Things
to Go Well

*Expectations
influence outcome.*

I have said that breast cancer is a game of chance. It is a game of chance, but you have more control over its outcome than you might think. There's a joker in the deck, and it can double the value of whatever hand you choose to play. What's more, you already hold it. It's your attitude....

A positive attitude will make everything you do to improve your chances of recovery more effective. In the end, it may prove to be more important than your choice of doctor or your choice of treatment. While most of us have grown up believing that the power to heal comes from outside of us—from doctors, drugs, and surgery—the truth is that while medical treatment comes from outside, healing comes from within.

As you and your doctor work together to restore your health, he will do his best to remove the cancer that is making you ill, but your body must do its own healing and reestablish its normal functions. Don't worry, it knows how. For all the progress medical science has made, it has taken only its first baby steps toward understanding how the human body rights itself when something throws it out of balance. You, on the other hand, were born knowing, not on a conscious level, but in the natural, encoded wisdom of every cell in your body.

Your active participation in your healing is important any time you are sick, but it is even more vital when you have an illness like breast cancer. Although we have gotten used to calling breast cancer a disease, this time your body is not the victim of some invading bacteria or virus. Your own cells have gone haywire, and for some reason your immune system, which is supposed to stop the wild growth of maverick cells, isn't doing its job. Your tumor is proof that your immune system is at least temporarily overwhelmed by fast-growing cancer cells. The goal of your medical treatment is to remove or greatly diminish the number of outlaw cells, so that your body can take back control and return to its normal operations, which include healing whatever damage has been done and preventing future problems.

Every human body is equipped with emergency powers for dealing with threats to its survival. Given some medical assistance and the right signals from you, *your* body will set its miraculous healing powers in motion and do all it can to put things right. How do you send it the right signals? By being positive and optimistic and letting it know you want your health back.

I'm not going to pretend that I know how a positive attitude jump-starts the body's healing mechanisms or a how defeatist attitude locks them down. I don't think anyone really knows. But there is plenty of evidence that attitude plays a major role in recovery from illness. Studies abound—some of which I have already mentioned—which prove that people who are upbeat and have a strong desire to return to health benefit more from medical treatment and recover more often than people who give up hope. Optimism doesn't guarantee recovery, of course, but even for those who don't recover, it makes a measurable difference. Patients with a positive attitude tend to live longer and feel better right up to the end than those who are negative.

In *To Be Alive,* oncologist Dr. Carolyn Runowicz notes, "through the years I've noticed anecdotally that my patients with a more positive attitude do seem to do better than those who have resigned themselves to die." [68] Later in the book she offers more solid evidence: "One cancer research team studied 69 women who had breast cancer, classifying their responses to illness: those who were feistier, who showed a fighting spirit, were twice as likely to survive five years as those who were into stoic acceptance or who felt hopeless about their future." [69]

Dr. Deepak Chopra, who in his medical practice and his best-selling books stresses the ability of the mind to marshal the body's natural healing powers, believes that attitude has a direct effect on body chemistry. "It is well documented that in a climate of negativity, the ability to heal is greatly reduced," he says in *Quantum Healing*. "Depressed people not only lower their immune response, for example, but even weaken their DNA's ability to repair itself." [70] I have to say that Chopra's detailed explanations of internal body chemistry went over my head, but his conclusion, like that of Dr. Runowicz and many other doctors, was clear. A positive attitude makes a difference in how a patient responds to treatment, and not a little difference—a very big difference.

As with computers and telephones, it's not important for us laymen to understand how this particular phenomenon works; we just need to know how to use it to improve our lives. From my own experience and observations I have concluded that it all comes down to expectations. Your body responds to your expectations, making what you think is going to happen actually happen much of the time. It may not be a very sophisticated theory, but once I realized its basic truth, a lot of things snapped into focus, and that's profound enough for me.

I predict that as you go through the testing and treatment that comes with breast cancer, if you expect to feel energetic and strong, you will. By the same token, if you expect to be miserable, uncomfortable, and depressed, you probably will be. Why would you want to do that to yourself?

I went in for my mastectomy surgery thinking I wouldn't have much pain afterward and would be back on my feet right away. I can't say why I thought that. Maybe it was wishful thinking, or my total lack of experience with surgery. Maybe it was because I was looking forward to the operation to finally end my months-long ordeal, or because I believed in my surgeon. I have a friend who fought and finally beat an advanced case of ovarian cancer, the disease that killed her mother. She pointed out to me one day that although we both were struggling with forms of cancer that had struck our mothers, I had a great psychological advantage because my mother had come out fine. While she was trying to quell her fears that she would share her mother's fate, I was planning for my healthy life after cancer.

Whatever their source, my positive expectations turned out to be true. No pain. No discomfort. No problem moving my arm. No excuse for the doctor to keep me in the hospital more than just overnight. A few days after surgery I was active and feeling fine, even while the surgical tubes still dangled from my chest.

Now, I'm not saying your experience will be the same as mine. You may go in for surgery expecting no negative aftereffects and still wake up to pain. If so, you can ask for medication to stop it. Actually, some form of pain medication will probably be right there anyway, just as my self-serve morphine was already attached to my IV, because the hospital staff expects you to have pain. If you trust that the medication will take care of your pain, it probably will. Research has shown that the effectiveness of drugs, too, is influenced by the patient's expectations.

In his book *Getting Well Again*, Dr. O. Carl Simonton reports on a study that divided patients with bleeding ulcers into two groups. The groups were given the same drug, but different expectations. The first group was told the drug was known to be effective, so they expected it to work. The second group was told the drug's effects were unknown, so they didn't know what to expect. After taking the drug, 70 percent of those in the first group improved significantly, but only 25 percent of those in the second group did. [71]

Although I had no pain from my mastectomy, I have certainly had pain at other times in my life, and I have observed that when you expect pain, it hates to let you down. Obviously, we all have experienced pain we didn't expect, but when you do expect it, you look for it and wait for it, and then when it arrives you focus on it, and that focus gives it power.

Dr. David Spiegel, a professor of psychiatry at the Stanford University School of Medicine, told journalist Bill Moyers, "You have to pay attention to pain for it to hurt." [72] I believe that is true of physical *and* emotional pain, both of which you may face during your time as a breast cancer patient and in the months and years that follow. No one can say what your individual experience will be like, but I feel safe in predicting that whatever happens will be a whole lot easier to handle if your attitude is positive and optimistic.

The Power of Belief

I think that as a society we greatly underestimate the power of belief. We may nod in agreement when a minister declares that faith can move mountains, but we don't really know how to apply that information to our lives. I wanted in this chapter to point to a number of examples from our popular culture to illustrate how if you believe in yourself you can accomplish amazing things. I came up with just one story, *The Little Engine That Could*, one of my favorite childhood books. Remember "I think I can, I think I can"? Surprised that I couldn't dredge up any other examples, I began to wonder, why was it so easy to come up with widely-known "helpless female" myths for chapter 8 and so hard to think of myths that illustrate the power of belief in oneself? The individual's power to accomplish what at first appears impossible seems not to be a theme our culture has chosen to emphasize, except when it comes to material success. I think we need someone to write some new stories for our common mythology.

While we're waiting, we can learn something about the power of belief from cultures other than our own. I found some stunning examples last summer, when I wasn't even looking for them. I was after some escapist vacation reading when I came across a copy of Wade Davis's *The Serpent and the Rainbow*. The cover blurb promised a tale of exotic adventure: "A Harvard scientist uncovers the startling truth about the secret world of Haitian voodoo and zombies." I was hooked. As I soon found out, Davis, a graduate student in ethnobotany, was sent to Haiti in 1982 to search for the botanical sources of drugs reportedly used to turn people into the walking dead. He gradually worked his way into the heart of the voodoo culture and actually succeeded in finding both zombies and the source of the drugs that "kill" and then revive them. He observed that although the drugs are real and powerful, the overriding reason they work is that the victims believe they work. "Clearly it is the victim's mind that mediates the sorcerer's curse and the fatal outcome," Davis says. "Fear, in other words, could initiate actual physiological changes that quite literally led to death." [73]

Davis was not surprised to find that the power of the drugs lies in the attitude of the person who takes them. It is the same, he says, with any drug, positive or negative. "This is what experts call the 'set and setting' of any drug experience," he explains. "*Set* in these terms is the individual's expectations of what the drug will do to him; *setting* is the environment—both physical and, in this case, social—in which the drug is taken." [74] In Haiti, people grow up believing that the voodoo priest and his drugs have supernatural power, and so they do.

The book brought back to my mind a vivid scene from the Australian film *The Last Wave*, in which an aboriginal elder kills a man by menacingly pointing a bone at him. My daughter was haunted by that scene for months afterward, unable to understand how the elder could kill a person without even touching him.

"The man's own fear killed him," I finally explained. "He believed he would die if that bone was pointed at him. When it happened, his terror caused him to collapse, probably of a heart attack."

We have been taught to look down on such happenings and the cultures in which they occur as primitive and bizarre. While we scoff, shamans in places like Haiti and Australia skillfully manipulate one of the most potent forces on earth—the power of the human mind to control the body—using it to cure far more often than to kill.

Because the power of belief to bring about physiological changes doesn't fit easily into the structure of Western medicine, it has been largely belittled and brushed aside here. Still, I'm sure you have come across it. American doctors refer to it— usually in a dismissive tone— as "the placebo effect."

Respect for the Placebo Effect

The few placebo studies that have been formally conducted in the United States have confirmed the awesome power of expectations. In one, cited by Caryle Hirshberg and Marc Ian Barasch in their book *Remarkable Recovery*, the control group in a chemotherapy study received infusions of mild salt water instead of drugs. Thirty percent lost all of their hair, because they believed they were getting chemo drugs and expected hair loss to be a side effect. [75]

In *Anatomy of an Illness*, Norman Cousins describes a number of other examples, including a study of ascorbic acid (vitamin C) as a cold preventive at the Mount Sinai Medical Center in New York. Participants who took placebos but thought they were getting vitamins had fewer colds than those who took vitamins but thought they were placebos. Cousins also cites a study of surgery patients in which a placebo was 77 percent as effective as morphine in stopping postoperative pain. [76]

Cousins concludes, as did Wade Davis, that the expectations with which a drug is taken powerfully influence its effect. He argues that there was a time when Western physicians knew this to be true, and relied upon it: "Respectable names in the history of medicine, like Paracelsus, Holmes and Osler, have suggested that the history of medication is far more the history of the placebo effect than of intrinsically valuable and relevant drugs." [77]

Although Western doctors today tend to belittle the placebo effect, there has been some progress in exploring the power of the mind over the body. With the assistance of biofeedback machines that do nothing more than measure their success, thousands of patients have learned to use their minds to change their body temperature, blood pressure, pulse rate, and other vital functions, and thus to control a variety of painful and dangerous conditions without drugs.

Perhaps the ultimate demonstration of the power of the mind to affect the body is hypnotism, once considered a nightclub act but now on its way to becoming an alternative form of medical treatment. I remember as a child hearing stories of the hypnotist who puts a subject in a trance and says he is going to touch her arm with a hot iron. He then touches her with a pencil, she shrieks, and a blister appears on the spot he touched. Subjects under hypnosis react physically to what they believe is happening. They can be made to feel pain when there is nothing to cause it, or not to feel pain when there is major cause. They can be cured of addictions, as my brother-in-law was cured of a long-time smoking habit in one session.

We have all run into situations of one kind or another that demonstrate the power of mind over matter. I have watched my daughter's soccer team look over their opponents before a game and decide they can't win. They then go out on the field and play miserably: missing kicks, running at half speed, and generally making their prophecy come true. On the other hand, I have seen them decide they're going to win, and go out and play like champs. They make happen what they expect to happen.

When we were looking for a private school for our daughter, my husband and I spoke with one headmaster about the widespread phenomenon of girls, once they reach a certain age, doing poorly in math and science. He told us he had grown up in Scotland and taught math there as a young man. Until he came to the U.S., he had never heard of girls doing worse than boys in those subjects. "Either American girls are different from girls in other countries," he said, "or what you have here is a self-fulfilling prophecy." The girls at his highly regarded school are expected to excel. Year after year they equal or outperform the boys in math and science. I know, because our daughter is one of them.

Doctor, What Should I Expect?

Knowing how we are all influenced by expectations—our own and those of the people in positions of authority around us—I can't help wondering how differently women with breast cancer would feel if doctors, for instance, assured us we would be fine, physically and psychologically, after a mastectomy. I wonder how much difference it would make in the way we respond to treatment if all women knew that the majority of those who get breast cancer come out of it okay, so we all have reason to be optimistic. I wonder what would happen if doctors actually told their patients that we can improve our chances significantly simply by adopting an optimistic, confident outlook.

I was encouraged recently to see one health-care organization doing just that, and I was especially pleased that it was my own HMO, Kaiser Permanente. Kaiser, an extraordinarily sensible operation, has for a while now been emphasizing the role patients play in their own health care. Every few months I get a members' magazine in the mail; it's called *Partners in Health.* In the Summer 1996 issue, Dr. David S. Sobel, Northern California Director of Patient Education, offered this unusual piece of medical advice: "Reaching for medication may not always be the best solution. If given time to work, your body is its own healer. Your brain has a built-in 'pharmacy' of healing mechanisms that are often safer and more effective than any drug." When you do take a drug, Sobel goes on to explain, it elicits two reactions. "One is determined by the chemical nature of the medication. The second is triggered by your beliefs and expectations concerning the medication. Every time you take a medication, you are swallowing not only a drug, but also your expectations and beliefs. The key to taking advantage of your internal pharmacy is to develop positive expectations."

I hope other health-care organizations and individual doctors are moving in the same direction, acknowledging the importance of expectations and encouraging patients to take a more active role in their own health care. I am afraid, however, that the change, if it is indeed coming, will take a long time. We cannot afford to wait for the professionals, nor do we need to. We can begin taking on more responsibility for our health care right now. We can change our attitudes from passive acceptance of both illness and treatment to active stimulation of our bodies' healing mechanisms and informed participation in choosing our therapies. It may sound like a major undertaking, especially for someone who is or may be seriously ill, but what could be a better use of our energies?

Recognizing Our Mythical Realities

Since our beliefs about ourselves and about medical care in general are at the heart of our expectations, they are the logical place to start. Although we think we know ourselves, I have come to believe that most of us, perhaps all of us, live in what I call "mythical realities." We have accepted as true a number of ideas about ourselves and the world that are actually myths, and we have allowed them to dictate our thoughts and actions. After a while it no longer matters that the basic concepts are untrue. The mythical reality has become our life.

If you look carefully, I think you will find some myths that are driving *you*. What beliefs is your body image based on? Do you believe, for instance, that there is a single standard of female beauty, compared with which you are too thin or too fat?

Do you believe men are attracted to women because of their breasts, and that no man would want you if you lost one?

Do you believe breast cancer is a death sentence?

Do you believe a woman who has breast cancer will be sick forever?

Do you believe if you talk to friends about your illness they won't want to be around you?

Do you believe sick people ought to stay at home and act like sick people?

Are you letting someone else's view of the world determine yours?

It isn't easy to recognize and reject your mythical reality, but it can be terribly important. As hard as it is for us as individuals, I think it is harder still for women as a group. We are constantly being manipulated by huge institutionalized myths that are all around us, on the airwaves, in books and magazines, in store windows, in conversations with friends who are as convinced as we are. Everyone is afraid to be the one who speaks out against a prevailing myth. And yet, seeing the truth and speaking it can make all the difference.

As children we chuckled at Hans Christian Andersen's story of the Emperor striding down the street in his new, imaginary clothes. The clever and treacherous tailors had declared them the most magnificent clothes ever made, and all the people in the kingdom acted as if it were so. No one had the courage to challenge the prevailing myth—until a child blurted out the truth. We need that child here today. We need to be that child.

I discovered when I was struggling with breast cancer that my true feelings were not what I was being told every woman feels. As soon as I recognized and accepted that fact, the myths began to crumble. If you make an effort to discover what you really feel—about your body, your health, your breasts—you too may find a new, more positive reality against which to measure the advice and expectations of others. With a clearer vision of who you are, you will be better able to choose the course of action that is right for you and feel the power and satisfaction of being an active participant in one of the most important episodes of your life.

Some doctors warn that once people realize their attitudes can influence their health, they may feel guilty that they "let themselves get sick" or have failed to cure themselves. Dr. David Sobel at Kaiser, while stressing the importance of a positive attitude, cautions that "an overzealous belief in 'mind over matter' can lead to damaging and unhealthy feelings of guilt." [78] Don't let yourself go from a feeling of helplessness to a belief that everything rests on your shoulders. A positive attitude can help the healing process tremendously, but it will not, by itself, protect you from cancer or cure it. It is one more tool in your personal health-care kit. It would be foolish to ignore it, but it is just as foolhardy to expect it to do every job on its own.

Resisting feelings of helplessness and fear is one of your most important responsibilities as a patient. There is no one right way to do it. Some women find their faith in the future is boosted by meditation or prayer. Others are energized by social activities or by self-expression through art, dance, or music. Whatever makes you feel strong and connected to the world around you will help to keep you positive and moving toward recovery.

We cannot always choose what will happen to us in our lives, but we can choose how we respond. We can be pessimistic or optimistic, passive or involved; we can allow breast cancer to overwhelm us or deal with it decisively and move on.

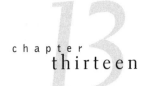

Trust Your Body's Ability to Heal

The human body is a miraculous healing machine.

Looking back on my own experience, it seems to me there are three distinct phases of breast cancer that have three different emotional levels and require three different types of coping. We have already talked about two of them. The first phase, discovery, lasts from the moment you or someone else discover a lump in your breast until you take the first test to determine its nature. Although it is a very intense, worry-filled time that calls for quick and deliberate action, it is usually mercifully short....

The second phase, testing and treatment, is also an intense time. Depending on the seriousness of your condition and the nature of the treatment you choose, it can last for many months or even years. It feels less frightening than the discovery phase because it is a time of abundant support. Besides attracting the concern of friends and family, during this phase you are surrounded by doctors and other medical professionals who keep your mind busy and your schedule full.

Sadly, some women—those with advanced metastatic breast cancer—never move beyond the second phase. The vast majority, however, do. For many, phase three, recovery and getting on with your normal life, is the most trying time of all. The shock of discovery and the intense focus of testing and treatment are past. The doctors have turned their attention to other patients. It's suddenly up to you and your body to finish the job. Phase three stretches from the day you complete treatment through all the rest of your life. It is punctuated by occasional medical checkups, but for the most part, you're on your own.

After long months of having doctors to tell you what to do and how you're going to feel, you suddenly feel you're facing the future alone. Expect to be filled with doubts and fear at first. Everyone is. You will probably wish you could continue to have doctors around you, overseeing each step you take on the road back to health. The fact is, however, like it or not, once you have completed treatment you have moved beyond the doctors' expertise. Like soldiers, doctors are trained for battle, not for rebuilding. The greatest expert in that field, in whose abilities you must now put your trust, is your own body.

I never thought about how much we take the incredible healing powers of our bodies for granted until I entered this final phase. If you are having trouble believing that you can bounce back and feel normal again after breast cancer, stop right now and think about all the miracles your body has already performed for you. Just in the course of living your life, you have undoubtedly injured yourself countless times. You have had scrapes and bruises and cuts, and they have all healed with very little intervention from you or anyone else. There have probably been times when you ate something unfit to eat, and your body knew immediately and heaved it back. Perhaps you have broken a bone, which needed only to be set back in its proper position for it to knit together again.

These are common events in all of our lives, and they are miracles. For all our scientific knowledge, doctors don't know how these everyday miracles happen, and can't make them happen. For all their years of study, medical researchers have not come up with an operation that can knit two parts of a broken bone together or a drug that can make a scraped elbow grow new skin. They don't need to, you may say; those things just happen automatically. Exactly. They happen because our bodies have an astounding ability and a powerful natural drive to heal themselves. They do it so often, so well, and so completely without fanfare that we hardly take notice of their amazing feats.

Over the years your body has given you a million reasons to trust its ability to heal itself. A 6-inch mastectomy incision across your chest is undeniably a bigger healing job than, say, a paper cut on your finger, but the difference is in its scale, not its essential nature. An incision is a cut, and so long as it was skillfully done, it's going to heal just fine. Radiation and chemotherapy are harder on a body than surgery alone, but you have recovered from burns in the past and from poisons of one kind or another that got into your system. If your treatments were extensive and the damage considerable, you will take longer to heal than someone who had surgery alone, but your body will push hard to reestablish its normal functions and vitality. Trust it, even when the going seems slow and rough.

Patience, Patient

○

I was astounded by how quickly my mastectomy incision healed. Two weeks after surgery, when the staples came out, the cut was already completely closed. I thought that would be all there was to it, but I guess that would have been too easy. While I knew my mastectomy was a good thing, all my body knew was that it had been injured. It immediately geared up to fix the damage, first pumping great quantities of fluid into the cavity where my breast had been to cushion the remaining tissue while it healed. Your body does the same thing when a new shoe rubs a raw spot on your foot or a hot oven shelf burns your finger. This wasn't a little blister, though; this was the whole left side of my chest. I was upset about it, until I saw how completely calm Dr. S. was. He said cheerfully that the fluid was a natural reaction; unnecessarily abundant perhaps, but natural. He'd just drain it out every few days until it stopped coming, however long it took. It took about three weeks.

Given all the emphasis these days on medical and especially surgical intervention, it was strangely reassuring to hear Dr. S. say he would simply drain and wait. During those weeks when he was unable to do much as a surgeon, he was most effective as a doctor. His impressive technical skills took a back seat to comforting conversation and common sense. He trusted my body to do its job, and he taught me to be patient and trust it too.

Your body, like mine, will work its own way back toward health. Perhaps your doctor will find little ways of helping it along (Dr. S. finally inserted a tube to make the draining constant), but essentially he, and you, will help most by just being patient.

I feel I should mention here that there are people who believe so strongly in their bodies' natural defenses and healing abilities that they choose to deal with their cancer without medical assistance. I am not one of them. I know my body can cope with colds and flu, bleeding cuts and nasty blisters, but when it came to cancer, I wanted the best professional help I could find. Still, I am intrigued by stories, some of them well documented, of people who, either by choice or because they were beyond medical help, went untreated and experienced so-called spontaneous remissions of cancer. I wish that instead of ignoring such cases, medical researchers would study them and perhaps discover the mechanisms that empower some people to eliminate tumors on their own. They may be rare cases, but I can't help feeling they are harboring a secret that could revolutionize our approach to cancer.

In the meantime, luckily, we don't have to understand how our inborn healing mechanisms work to benefit from them. We just have to trust them to do their job, and avoid doing anything to interfere with them. Whatever condition your body is in after breast cancer treatment, it is going to do all it can to bring you back to normal, simply because that's what healthy bodies do. Perhaps you don't think of your body as healthy anymore, but if your treatment has eliminated all detectable signs of cancer, chances are good that you are indeed healthy again. Your body may be damaged by the treatments it has undergone, but it is no longer sick. It will do its best to repair itself, as it has always done in the past, and it will do so amazingly quickly if you help it along.

Setting the Stage for Healing

We have already discussed improving your eating and exercise habits, giving up smoking, and keeping a positive attitude. There is one more thing you need to do to help your body heal, and that is to provide as stress-free an environment as you possibly can.

Stress is one of the omnipresent evils of our fast-paced lifestyle. It causes illness and interferes with healing. At some level, we all know that stress is bad for us, but most of us think of stress as something we're stuck with. In fact, there are many ways of reducing stress, but it takes a bit of refocusing, especially for breast cancer patients. During our months of testing and treatment, and of facing an uncertain future, most of us have gotten so used to stress that it feels normal to us. The first step we have to take, which in some ways is the hardest, is simply learning to see where stress is coming from. We are by no means the only people who have problems with this.

Recently, a male friend and I sat at the dinner table talking about the psoriasis that plagues us both. I said I am certain mine is stress-related; it flares up whenever I am under a lot of pressure. He said he has never noticed a connection to stress. His case was in full bloom that night, but he said he hadn't been under any stress at all. His wife agreed. "His life is really stress-free," she said. I stared at them in disbelief. Not ten minutes earlier, my friend had been complaining that he still had pain from the extraction of several wisdom teeth a week before. A week of constant pain sounded like a stressful situation to me. What's more, when I had called to invite them to dinner about two weeks before, his wife had said he couldn't come to the phone because he was so upset by a computer problem he was having. He had been tearing his hair out in frustration for three days, she said.

I don't know why so many of us deny, or are unable to see, that situations like these are stressful. Perhaps we think we should be able to tolerate pain and handle tough problems without help and without getting ruffled. The fact is that in most cases we can't. Stress is a normal response to difficulties and discomfort. Usually there is something you can do to reduce the stress, but first you have to acknowledge that it's bothering you.

The Pros and Cons
of a Hospital Stay

For me, being in the hospital was extremely stressful. I know a hospital is supposed to be a peaceful, nurturing place. I found it to be just the opposite. Once I was out of surgery and installed in my tiny hospital room, all I wanted was to go home. The bed was uncomfortable. I had to call a nurse to unhook me from some machine every time I needed to go to the bathroom. And the constant drone of other people's televisions hung in the air. Once the aftereffects of anesthesia wore off, I felt fine physically, but I felt trapped. I keep reading that breast cancer activists want hospitals to keep patients two nights after a mastectomy. That would have been horrible for me.

I had fortified myself against the inevitable hours of boredom in the hospital by bringing a portable CD player and my favorite music—loud, rollicking rock 'n' roll. As soon as I was fully awake, I put on the headphones and I was on a bright oasis. I could feel the energy flowing back into my body.

When a knot of young doctors arrived at my bedside early on the morning after my surgery, I was wearing my headset and humming along with Bruce Springsteen. The doctors commented on how cheerful I looked. They also declared that all my vital signs were surprisingly good. At about 7 o'clock Dr. S. appeared and said I looked too healthy to be in the hospital. "Go home," he said. It was music to my ears. As soon as he walked out, I called Jay. "Come get me," I said jubilantly.

I know everyone doesn't share my impatience with hospitals. You may like staying and resting for a few days after surgery. If so, fine. But if the hospital is a source of stress for you, as soon as you feel well enough to go home, let the doctors know that you want to be released.

Go Easy on Yourself

Of course, there is going to be plenty of stress waiting at home. If you expect too much of yourself at first, you're sure to get frustrated. Everyone is tired after major surgery, both from the ordeal itself and from the aftereffects of anesthesia. So take it easy, especially in the first couple of weeks. Don't rush to return to work. Don't feel obligated to have visitors if you don't feel ready. And, for heaven's sake, let the housework go. It will still be there when you're feeling more energetic. If you feel tired, which you will most days, take a nap. A nap is a luxury. Take advantage. Take two. Don't feel guilty; enjoy it.

If you've had a mastectomy, you'll have the added stress of tubes and bottles dangling from your chest. I hated those bottles. They kept me from sleeping on my stomach and made my every move feel awkward. I was able to partially come to terms with them by strapping on my fanny pack and shoving them inside. Still, I let them become a source of worry in a way that, in retrospect, was foolish.

The breast care coordinator had told me the fluid in the bottles should lessen each day, and that it had to reach a certain low level

before my doctor would take out the tubes. Every time I emptied the
bottles I carefully measured and recorded the amount of fluid, as I'd
been instructed, and worried that the flow wasn't slowing down
enough. I grew more and more tense as the day of my follow-up
appointment approached, desperately wanting the annoying tubes out
and frustrated that the fluid wasn't lessening. The process that was
going on in my chest was beyond my control and I knew it, but that
didn't stop me from obsessing on it. I took my carefully kept record
with me to my postsurgery appointment, feeling defeated and doomed
to another week of those awful tubes. Dr. S. didn't even look at my
notes. He gently removed my bandages, then unceremoniously
yanked the tubes from my chest. He told me he didn't care about the
fluid flow; he thought leaving the tubes in was more of a danger.

That incident made me realize how much energy you can waste
focusing on something that turns out not to matter. Since then, I've
tried to relax and take things as they come, especially the ones I can't
change anyway.

Body Language

If you learn to "listen" to your body, it will tell you when it is struggling
under too much stress. Its language, which you must learn to interpret,
is one of symptoms.

My body communicates its distress to me mainly through my skin.
I had my first outbreak of psoriasis when I was 13. I was 18 and in college when I began suspecting that flare-ups were connected to stress. I
owe that insight to my freshman roommate, a flashy young woman
who took great pleasure in making my drab life miserable. She tor-
tured me regularly with little tricks like locking me out of our room
when I went down the hall to the bathroom, and putting up the shade

after I was asleep so a street lamp would shine in my eyes. She did a lot more serious things, not to me, that got her expelled at the end of the second semester. By then psoriasis was rampant on every part of my body and I was sure that living with her was the reason.

Since then I've looked to see what's going on in my life whenever my skin erupts. A strained relationship, frustrations at work, and financial woes have all translated to patchy scales somewhere on my body. The most amazing demonstration of my stress-skin connection occurred when a friend who had left California to go to medical school came to visit with a man she was dating. I found this man extraordinarily attractive, and as the three of us sat in my living room talking, I fantasized about being with him, imagining his hand touching my breast. The thought was simultaneously exciting and scary. That evening when I undressed, I found a new patch of psoriasis on my breast, right where I had envisioned him touching me.

I used to hate my outbreaks of psoriasis, but I slowly learned to appreciate them as helpful messages from my body. Now, instead of responding to them with anger, I respond with introspection, trying to pinpoint the source of stress and see if there is some way to eliminate or at least reduce it. I've found ointments that help to clear the affected skin, but only dealing with the underlying cause stops further eruptions.

My body has a couple of other ways it signals discomfort. Whenever I get nervous, I get diarrhea. I'm not going to stop meeting people or appearing at events that make me nervous, so in this case I concentrate on dealing with the symptom. I carry a supply of Pepto-Bismol, which allows me to push on through.

There's no way to stave off my other stress symptom. Just before every emotionally charged occasion in my life, from my bas mitzvah to my mastectomy, I have gotten my period, regardless of where I happened to be in my monthly cycle. I've come to expect it and, as annoying as it is, I accept it. These are my body's stress signals. Other people have different signals.

I once had a roommate who was a minister and told me about a minister friend of his who stuttered whenever he was under a lot of stress. Stuttering can be a major problem for a clergyman, and this man was extremely upset whenever it happened. Eventually, though, he came to see it as a blessing. It was a sign he couldn't overlook that warned him when he needed to slow down.

What are your symptoms of stress? Learn to recognize them, and you will have a dependable gauge of the pressure you are putting on your body. Once you are aware that your stress level has gotten too high, you can begin to do something to bring it back down, whether that means getting help with a problem, or withdrawing from a relationship, or simply taking time out for a walk or a relaxing bath. The trick is not to ignore your body's stress signals or try to suppress them with drugs, but to appreciate them for the red flags they are.

Reframing Your Situation

Taking something you're used to thinking of as negative, like psoriasis or a headache or a stiff neck, and turning it into something positive just by changing the way you look at it is called "reframing." It is a helpful technique for more than just dealing with stress. You can help your healing process along and transform your recuperation into a powerful growing experience by choosing to see this final phase of your breast cancer experience as positive rather than negative—as a time full of change and opportunity, rather than a frustratingly slow return to where you were before. Life after breast cancer has some tough moments—nobody can deny that—but if you want it to be, it can be a wonderful time. While your body heals, you have the perfect opportunity to redirect your life. Everyone is going to be expecting you to be different anyway, so why not take advantage?

If there is ever going to be a time when you have the freedom to focus on yourself, this is it. Don't think of yourself as unlucky because you've had breast cancer; focus on the opportunity you now have to change. As you start eliminating the sources of stress from your life, watch your body respond with higher energy and signs of returning health.

A word of warning: Don't make the mistake of setting deadlines for your recuperation. Your body is on its own schedule, and you have no way of knowing what that schedule is. You may heal faster or slower than other women in similar situations. Setting a timeline is setting yourself up for disappointment. Instead, celebrate your progress when it seems swift, and when it's slow, be patient and trust your body. After all, it's the final results that count, not how long it takes to get there.

I learned about the different timetables of women's bodies when I gave birth to my daughter. Several friends were pregnant at the same time I was, and we compared notes every step of the way. It was the first pregnancy for all of us, and we didn't know what to expect, so we tried to learn from each other. My friend Julie was out in front of the pack, about three months ahead of me. I intently watched her progress. When her time came to deliver, she popped out a baby boy in four hours flat. I thought that was great and was looking forward to doing the same.

Well, my baby wasn't so anxious to leave her comfortable internal environment. As soon as my water broke, on a sunny Saturday afternoon, Jay and I rushed to the hospital, and spent 27 ½ grueling hours there before Rebecca finally emerged. Julie could have delivered seven babies in the time it took me to push out just one. But, you know, we both had healthy babies. Today they're both making their mark on the sixth grade, and it doesn't make a bit of difference that one was born faster than the other. Everyone's body is different; there's no point in comparing them. Whether it's childbirth or recovering from breast cancer, it's the final result, not how long it takes to get there, that counts.

In a way, the journey back to health that is the third and final phase of breast cancer is never really over. It is a journey, yes, with a destination, but at the same time it is the rest of your life and every step along the way is its own experience. Breast cancer has forced you to take a detour, but now you're back on the road. If you let yourself get too focused on a distant goal, you'll miss all the good things along the way.

When I was a kid, I would sit in the back seat of my parents' car and ask a million times, "Are we there yet?" All I could think about was getting to the friend's house or the hotel we were aiming for. I don't think I saw much of the countryside outside the car windows.

After breast cancer, some women likewise set their sights on a point way down the road, a future date when they will believe that they are well again. Ten years is a common choice, and one encouraged by the way survival statistics are reported. If I make it for ten years, they say, then I'll be safe; then I can breathe a sigh of relief and get on with my life. Meanwhile, their lives are rolling by, almost unnoticed.

Let the statisticians worry about the five-year marks and ten-year marks. Set your sights on enjoying every day as it comes and goes.

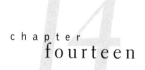

Appreciate
the New You

*A one-breasted
body isn't ugly,
just different.*

I reacted emotionally to many parts of my breast cancer experience, but the part I reacted to most strongly, and most angrily, was being pressured to have breast reconstruction....

I think it is insulting to suggest that a woman who loses a breast to cancer can no longer feel like a "whole woman." This bit of nonsense has been repeated so often it has begun, for many women, to sound like truth. It is a cultural lie, every bit as destructive and debilitating as the lies that have convinced millions of American women they must be thin as a rail to be attractive.

I am very glad I rejected Dr. S.'s recommendation of breast reconstruction and left my postmastectomy body unaltered. To those with doubts I can honestly report that after four years I am still very much a woman. In fact, I am more of a woman—more productive professionally, more active sexually, more self-assured, a better wife and mother, healthier, and a good deal happier than I was when I had two breasts. Nothing bad or embarrassing has happened to me because of my lopsidedness. Nothing.

To a surprising extent, the emotional crisis everyone says comes with losing a breast is a fraud. It is a manufactured phenomenon, like the assorted "female crises" described by Susan Faludi in *Backlash*: "From 'the man shortage' to 'the infertility epidemic' to 'female burnout' to 'toxic day care,' these so-called female crises have had their origins not in the actual conditions of women's lives but rather in a closed system that starts and ends in the media, popular culture, and advertising—an endless feedback loop that perpetuates and exaggerates its own false images of womanhood." [79] The impact of these imagined crises comes not from the experience they claim to focus on, but from the self-destructive panic response they spawn. If you believe that losing your breast will ruin your self-confidence or your social life, it very well may. If, on the other hand, you are skeptical and trust your own experience rather than the dire predictions of others, you may find, as I did, that it doesn't affect you much at all.

Sizing Up the Changes in Your Body

There is no denying that your body will be different after mastectomy. I call it a new body, but it will actually be a new version of your same body, and it will function the same as it always has or even better because it will be healthier. The one thing your body will no longer be able to do is nurse a baby on the side that has had surgery. Since breast cancer is largely a postmenopausal disease, that's not usually a problem. If you earn your living as a wet nurse, mastectomy is going to disrupt your life. Otherwise you'll be fine. The only significant change will be in your appearance.

Ah, your appearance. Advertising agencies and the popular culture machine have spent years trying to convince you that your value as a woman depends on your appearance matching their selected standard of beauty. Have they succeeded? Do you find it hard to believe that you will be the same attractive, lovable, capable woman after mastectomy as before?

If you are considering reconstruction, I urge you to take your time and think the matter through carefully before you commit yourself. No matter what you've been told, once you've undergone mastectomy you are not going to get your breast back. Only God can make a tree, and only an adolescent female body can make a breast. It is important to understand that a reconstructed breast is at best an approximation, an artist's conception of a female breast. A very good one can fool people into thinking you still have your breast (so long as you don't take your clothes off), but it isn't a functioning or feeling breast, and it's not going to fool you.

Reconstruction is a harsh and simplistic physical solution to a complicated psychological and social problem. It is harsh because it requires a woman who has just undergone major surgery, to say nothing of facing a threat to her life, to submit to several more rounds of surgery, with all the attendant risks, when there is no medical reason to do so. It is simplistic because it equates the surface problem—a woman's missing breast—with the deep psychological and emotional causes of her pain and imagines that by patching the first it can cure the second.

Many surgeons, both male and female, seem to assume that every patient will want an artificial breast installed after mastectomy. The assumption is so widespread, in fact, that in many doctors' minds mastectomy is linked with reconstruction as one procedure. Women with breast cancer are routinely presented with a choice between lumpectomy with radiation and mastectomy with reconstruction.

In my case, reconstruction was not offered as an opportunity; it was presented as an obligation, and I had to fight to avoid it. Mastectomy and reconstruction are sometimes even performed during the same operation, with an oncological and a cosmetic surgeon working side by side. I find this double-barreled procedure disturbing because it doesn't give women who are caught up in the trauma of breast cancer the time to weigh their alternatives. Many women who wait to consider reconstruction after they've healed from mastectomy decide that their bodies are fine and don't need an artificial breast after all.

Reconstruction Choices

In recent years, the problems with silicone breast implants have led to new approaches to breast reconstruction. Most reconstruction patients these days choose either an implant filled with saline solution or a new "breast" constructed out of flesh moved from elsewhere on the body. There are, of course, hazards connected with both methods, and neither guarantees the result will look right. As is the case with breast enlargement surgery, implants often need to be replaced after a time. For that reason, many surgeons favor using a woman's own tissue for reconstruction, using one of two basic approaches.

The differences between the two are in where the tissue for the artificial breast comes from and how it is moved. [80] With the "pedicle flap" procedure, tissue from a nearby location such as the abdomen or back is stretched to the chest while remaining attached to its natural location. As Dr. Susan Love describes it, the surgeon makes a tunnel and moves the tissue through it. The problem, she says, is that "we have to disturb all the tissue en route, so we're disturbing a lot of your body surface. What this means is that you'll have a lot of long-term complications that aren't terribly serious but can be pretty uncomfortable." Some of the complications she mentions are stiffness, pain, loss of strength, and, of course, scars.

The second approach is the "free flap" procedure, in which tissue is cut away from the donor body part and planted in the chest area. The operation, which includes sewing blood vessels together under a microscope, is very complicated. It takes five to eight hours, according to Love, and is followed by a hospital stay of four to seven days. "It's certainly an ordeal to go through," she says, "and the ordeal continues for a time, in a milder form—you'll probably end up getting a second operation for final touch-ups, and to make a nipple if you want one." Some women, I gather, don't bother to go back for the nipple, which is made from tissue from elsewhere on the body and then tattooed to add color.

So what exactly does an artificial breast, with or without nipple added, look like? The answer is that they vary greatly, and you should insist that any cosmetic surgeon you're considering show you pictures of the full range of his results, not just the ones he likes best.

The ones I saw in a plastic surgeon's slide show at a women's health seminar were unattractive, to say the least. Worse by far were the scars on the parts of the body from which the building materials were taken. One patient I particularly remember had had tissue removed from her stomach area. An enormous scar swooped from one hip all the way to the other. The women in the audience around me gasped at the sight.

"It is a big scar," the plastic surgeon conceded. "But it's worth it."

I have tried, especially since that seminar, to understand why women have breast reconstruction. I am lost. If your goal is to feel well physically after mastectomy, allowing your incision to heal naturally is obviously better than undergoing several more surgeries to have a bag of salt water or silicone planted in your chest or have it stuffed with a pound of your own flesh dragged or cut from somewhere else. If the idea is to look more normal, I don't see much advantage in a scarred, obviously artificial breast, even a nicely shaped one, especially if it comes with big, ugly scars on your stomach or buttocks or wherever. Such a "breast" may look natural when you're fully clothed, but the only people who really care about how your breasts look and feel—you and your lover—are going to see them naked. I have heard women say they chose reconstruction because they were afraid a flat chest and mastectomy scar would be constant, unpleasant reminders of their cancer ordeal. It seems to me the artificial, unfeeling breast, multiple scars, and pain and discomfort that come with reconstruction would be far worse reminders.

The Rise of Cosmetic Surgery

On the other hand, I have no trouble at all understanding why cosmetic surgeons are enthusiastic about breast reconstruction. It is a huge moneymaker in one of the fastest-growing medical specialties. In *To Dance with the Devil*, Karen Stabiner reports that one UCLA surgeon's fee for breast reconstruction was $14,000. [81] That's in addition to hospital charges and other related costs. It's a lot of money for a few hours of work.

Cosmetic surgery is a fascinating hybrid of medicine and fashion. It is the blatantly materialistic offshoot of plastic surgery, an admirable medical specialty that helps restore the bodies of burn and accident victims and correct some of the more flagrant mistakes of nature. Today's new breed of cosmetic surgeon focuses not on the ravages of disease or disaster, but on bruised and vulnerable egos. They alter the tummies, buttocks, chins, necks, noses, and eyelids of people, mostly women, who want desperately to be more attractive. They "resurface" skin and suck away fat. And they build new breasts and redesign existing ones.

"Breast enlargement surgery … is the second most frequently performed plastic surgery procedure on women," one of the regular ads in my local newspaper declares. "Breast reduction surgery is the most frequent operation I perform on the breast," says another. They make breasts bigger, they make them smaller. They lift sagging breasts and reposition nipples. They allure with fantasies and promise miracles. Their ads are adorned with photos of born-beautiful young women, naked or scantily clothed. "A plastic surgeon is like a sculptor," one ad announces. "Finding the perfect one is an art." It is an ad for a cosmetic surgery phone referral service, copyrighted, appropriately, by a company called Profitable Practices, Inc.

I think there are legitimate reasons for breast surgery, especially size reduction for women whose large breasts can cause back and shoulder problems and considerable physical pain. I also think if women with lots of money and insecurities want to have themselves surgically reshaped every now and then, that's their business. But I strongly object to women with breast cancer being pressured into such physically and psychologically dangerous territory. In *Catch-22*, one of Joseph Heller's characters says, "When I look up, I see people cashing in. I don't see heaven or saints or angels. I see people cashing in on every decent impulse and every human tragedy." [82] It bothers me to see people cashing in on breast cancer.

It bothers me and frightens me to see cosmetic surgery becoming commonplace. How did we arrive at the place where women have their bodies cut and rearranged and consider it normal? Author Susan Faludi traces the explosion of cosmetic surgery to 1983 when, she says, the American Society of Plastic and Reconstructive Surgeons decided their lagging business needed more customers and set out to do something about it. As Faludi describes it in *Backlash*, the organization "launched a 'practice enhancement' campaign, issuing a flood of press releases, 'pre- and post-op photos,' and patient 'education' brochures and videotapes. They billed 'body sculpturing' as safe, effective, affordable—and even essential to women's mental health." They zeroed in, especially, on women with small breasts. "'There is a body of medical information that these deformities [small breasts] are really a disease,' a statement issued by the society asserted; left uncorrected, flat-chestedness causes 'a total lack of well-being.'" [83]

In a realistic society, women would have gotten a good laugh from such a statement, but our culture is not based on reality, at least not when it comes to women's bodies. The campaign was successful, and the rush to breast implants was on, despite the physical dangers and decidedly mixed results. (According to Faludi, in at least 20 percent of the cases, repeat surgery was required to remedy pain, infection, blood clots, or implant ruptures, and a 1987 study in the *Annals of Plastic Surgery* reported that the implants failed as much as 50 percent of the time and had to be removed.) [84] In 1995, in their book *What Every Woman Should Know*, doctors Lila and Robert Nachtigall estimated that some two million American women had already had breast implants [85] — most of them healthy women, at least when they started out.

Fashion Becomes Medicine

As the overall breast-implant craze grew, the idea of rebuilding breasts for mastectomy patients also spread. Roberta Altman notes in *Waking Up, Fighting Back: The Politics of Breast Cancer* that in 1981 only about 20,000 American women had undergone breast reconstruction following a mastectomy. By 1985 (two years after the plastic surgeons' campaign) the number jumped to about 98,000, and by 1992, to 200,000. Still, Altman reports, according to FDA figures, in 1992 nearly two million women with mastectomies had not had reconstruction. [86]

Since then, the pace appears to have picked up dramatically. Dr. Carolyn Runowicz estimated in her 1995 book *To Be Alive* that more than half of new mastectomy patients were opting for reconstruction. [87] Other sources I have seen say the number is a bit below half. What, besides the obvious advertising blitz for cosmetic surgery, is pushing so many women toward reconstruction?

One major factor, I believe, is that oncological surgeons are recommending it more often and more forcefully to their patients. The cosmetic surgeons have managed to convince not only women, but their fellow doctors as well, that reconstruction is a psychological quick fix for the trauma of breast cancer. Perhaps surgeons are susceptible to the idea because they are so used to the practice of replacing lost body parts with artificial ones. Lost or damaged arms, legs, and hips are routinely replaced. The big difference is that the purpose of those replacements is to restore function, not appearance. Doctors who champion reconstruction ignore the fact that a substitute breast does not restore either function or feeling. It serves no medical purpose whatsoever. There is not a single thing a woman can do with an artificial breast that she cannot do without it, and that includes attracting lovers.

Of course, doctors don't tell us we need to have breast reconstruction to restore function. They tell us we need it to restore our self-image. Dr. S. told me, with great conviction and sincerity, that women don't heal well psychologically without it. I think by now he has reconsidered, at least in my one case. At my last checkup he marveled, "You look so healthy."

The weakness of the psychological argument for reconstruction is that it is based on a totally false premise: the assumption that women are not strong enough or flexible enough to adjust to a missing breast. Most of the women I know are very strong. They are intelligent, capable people who cope with difficult challenges every day. They simultaneously raise children, have active careers, maintain efficient households, are wives, volunteer workers, and pleasant, stimulating company. I find it hard to think of them as incapable of facing the realities of their health problems. If women have problems with psychological healing after mastectomy, it surely has less to do with any inherent weakness on their part than with the belittling advice they get from their trusted doctors and the negative expectations of those around them.

Women today are constantly being told that our breasts are the essence of our being, not only by those whose profits depend on our feelings of inadequacy, but by a wide range of well-meaning people who have been convinced that it is so. It is particularly depressing to hear strong, successful women, whom many of us look to as role models, reciting the mantra of the essential breast. In her book *To Dance with the Devil*, journalist Karen Stabiner ably documents "the new war on breast cancer." She focuses on Dr. Susan Love, whose strength and determination she obviously admires, but when she turns to the women who were Love's patients, she laments, "No matter what a woman did about her breast cancer, there was always the other issue: how she felt about her breasts. They were her vanity, her sex life, her motherhood, an outward symbol of an attractive and useful self." [88]

At least Stabiner acknowledges that the breast is "an outward symbol" of something within. Nurse Suzanne Zahrt Murphy, who has cared for, and presumably about, numerous mastectomy patients, is unfortunately more typical of the women who are speaking out on the subject of breast cancer. She confuses the symbol of womanhood with the real thing. Mastectomy, she wrote in the *San Francisco Chronicle*, is "removal of a body part that says you are a woman....Today you are a woman. Tomorrow, no matter how you try to cheer yourself, or become defiant, or stick to a 'scientific' attitude—that the cancer must be removed—you are going to be, says a voice inside your head (society's voice), half a woman.... you are giving up what you so anxiously waited for as a girl: breast/womanhood/desirability/mystical femininity." [89] Boy, am I glad she wasn't my post-op nurse.

Every once in a while, a voice is raised that contradicts such blind breast worship and sets straight some misconceptions about life after breast cancer. I wish every woman worried about losing a breast would read author Roberta Altman's description of her experience. "When I had the mastectomy," Altman writes, "I was living with a man. I couldn't conceive of Dave's loving me any less because I had just one breast. I was right. He was supportive and loving,...our sexual life continued as usual." A few years later they broke up and Altman began seeing other men. Worried about how they would react to her lopsidedness, she avoided intimate relationships until she started getting close to one particular man. After considerable hesitation and with great trepidation, she told him she had had a mastectomy. "So?" he replied. She burst into tears. "Did I say something wrong?" the bewildered man asked.

Altman continues, "He had no way of knowing that he was the first postmastectomy man I'd been with and that for months I'd been worrying what I'd say, how I'd say it, and what kind of response I'd get. As time passed and I had other relationships, I found that his reaction was typical. It seemed that my missing breast was more important to me than to the men I was seeing." [90]

I am convinced that the men Altman encountered are not unusual. Most men really don't care if a woman they find attractive has lost a breast. They are not as shallow as we think. It is our own hang-up on appearance, not theirs, that is driving us crazy.

Linda Dackman was young, attractive, and popular when she developed breast cancer and had a mastectomy. In her heart-wrenching book *Up Front*, she describes how her focus on appearance pushed her into breast reconstruction. "I was young enough and single enough that my whole emotional future seemed connected to how my body looked," she writes. "Although I probably would have denied it, I sought this operation with the vague hope that my physical and psychological transformation would be complete through the medical manipulation of skin, muscle, and implant. But that was not possible. At best, when I woke up after reconstruction, I felt married to a stranger. And it was not merely occupying my bed; it was permanently embedded in my body!" Dackman's disappointed evaluation of her reconstructed breast was that it was "no better than a flattened nippleless mound of dirt sitting on my chest wall.... So instead of the moment of transformation I had hoped for, reconstruction left me poised in a love/hate relationship with my body." [91]

I remember thinking, as I put down Dackman's book, *Why should this bright, creative, talented woman have to suffer so? Why was her self-image so attached to her breasts when she had so many other more important things going for her?* Dackman's insecurities, and Altman's, can be traced, I think, to our distorted cultural image of what men and women are like and what we want from each other. The popular image of the American woman, as seen in movies, on television, and in magazines, is someone eager to please but terminally insecure. No matter how successful she is in other parts of her life, she is constantly focused on her looks because she knows the only way for a woman to be happy is to snare a good-looking man. The media's American man is also insecure, though he's better at hiding it. He is sex-driven; chooses women according to their looks, especially their breast size; and expects them to shape, paint, and dress themselves to please him. In real life most people, both women and men, are better and smarter than that.

Talk It Over

The first step every woman should take before considering breast reconstruction is to talk to her partner. I imagine female partners, having breasts of their own, are not as intrigued by them, or as focused on them, as some men are. What surprised me, and may surprise you, was discovering that not all men are as hung up on breasts as we think they are. If you are thinking of reconstruction because you think your man, present or future, will reject you if you have just one breast, chances are you are underestimating him. I have asked a lot of men if they would feel any different about their wife or lover if she lost a breast, and not a single one has said yes. Most of them, in fact, looked at me like I was crazy to even ask. Real men are not like the men you see in movies and magazines.

Ask your lover to tell you frankly if he (or she) will love you or desire you any less after mastectomy. The answer may resolve your doubts and solve your imagined problem right then and there. If your lover tells you it's your health that's important, not your appearance, and you don't believe it, then perhaps the psychological problem is yours.

Now, there are men who, even after they know a woman well, focus most of their attention on how she looks, and you may have ended up somehow with one of them. Such men—arrested adolescents, one of my male friends calls them—are incapable of seeing the woman behind the breasts. If you are with a man like that, reconstruction will not change him. He will be as shallow and self-centered after your cosmetic surgery as before. The most important question to ask yourself, if you are with such a man, is not whether you should have reconstructive surgery, but why you stay with someone who values your looks above your health.

Some men who appear thick-headed and sexist are actually just immature and can be jolted into a growth spurt if they are challenged. To find out if your man is hopelessly mired in adolescent fantasies or is capable of achieving adulthood, you have to talk to him. I know this is hard, but it can change your life, and his. Tell him you appreciate him for the complete person he is and you want him to feel the same about you. Tell him his focus on your breasts makes you feel like he sees you as just a body. Tell him you didn't ask to have breast cancer, but it happened, and to handle it, both of you are going to have to grow up.

I'm not an expert in this area, but I suspect that a little shock to the ego may help move some men who are badly stuck but still capable of coming around. I sometimes wonder what would happen if a woman being pressured by her man to have reconstructive surgery were to say to him, "I understand, dear, that you liked my body the way it used to be. You know, I really liked yours the way it used to be too. Your slim waist, your flat stomach, your beautifully muscled abdomen, back, and arms, your thick blond (brown, red) hair. I understand why you want me to have my old body back, and I'm sure you can see why I would love you to have yours. I need my energy to heal from cancer right now, so why don't you go to the cosmetic surgeon first and have your body reconstructed? Then, when I'm feeling stronger, I'll go." Would he be appalled at the idea of going through surgery to restore his former shape? Why, then, shouldn't you?

Even if a conversation doesn't change either of your viewpoints, it should help you to see who is having a problem accepting your post-mastectomy body—you or him—and which of you needs help to adjust. In many cases, it will turn out to be both of you.

I don't understand why psychological counseling is not offered as a regular part of breast cancer treatment and follow-up care. The emotional turmoil many women with breast cancer go through can be even more damaging than the disease itself. A surgery department receptionist at the hospital told me one day, with a chilling mixture of sadness and frustration in her voice, that she has seen women come through the office who chose to let cancer kill them rather than face the loss of a breast. On another day, a nurse escorting me to an examination room spoke of the many women she had talked to who were convinced that after their mastectomies their husbands would no longer want them. She shook her head in dismay, but didn't offer any suggestion for how to change the situation.

I think the answer is obvious. You treat a patient with a psychological problem by calling in an expert on psychological problems. A woman who is having trouble dealing with the loss of a breast doesn't need a phony replacement breast; she needs someone to help her see her value as a human being, with or without a breast.

If you are upset about losing your breast and your surgeon offers to refer you to a plastic surgeon, ask for a referral to a psychotherapist instead. Be prepared for the surgeon's negative response at first. It may take some talking to convince him that you want to come to terms with your situation emotionally before you start fiddling around with your body. Surgeons are used to solving problems with a scalpel, and many of them are uncomfortable discussing the emotional aspects of illness, especially an illness with sexual implications. Taking time out for therapy will not affect your ability to have breast reconstruction even if you decide later that that is really what you want. Even strong advocates of reconstructive surgery agree that it can be done at any time, even years after your cancer surgery. On the other hand, once you have had reconstruction you can't easily reverse it. You owe it to yourself to be sure before you take so drastic and permanent a step.

If your doctor won't help you find a good therapist, find one yourself. I suggest you look for one who specializes in women's attitudes toward their bodies. A therapist who works with clients with eating disorders such as anorexia, bulimia, and compulsive eating understands the powerful role body image plays in women's lives. She will understand the pain you are feeling.

Take a few months, or longer if you need to, for counseling. Put off any decision about your outward appearance; instead, search inside of you for the true source of your womanhood. You may be amazed by what you find.

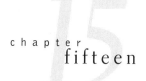

Sex Is in Your Head

Losing a breast doesn't have to affect your sex life.

What will happen to your sex life if you lose a breast to cancer? That depends entirely on your attitude. For women who consider themselves as attractive and sexual as ever, sexual relationships go on as before, or improve. For women who decide their sex life is over, it's over, or soon will be....

Despite our culture's insistence on equating sexiness with appearance, the truth is that sexiness is an attitude, not a body shape. People of all sizes and shapes enjoy sex. If a perfect body were a prerequisite, the human race would have died out long ago. There is just one basic requirement for sexual attractiveness—a positive attitude about yourself, your partner, and sex itself.

We women are constantly being given reasons to feel negative about ourselves, and most of us judge ourselves harshly. We have been taught to scrutinize our bodies daily and treat even a minor, temporary flaw like a pimple or a bad haircut as a disaster. How in the world are we supposed to deal with a missing breast? I'll tell you how. By accepting it for what it is: the mark left by our encounter with cancer and our triumph over it. Some women actually come to see their missing breast as a positive thing. I have.

What does a missing breast really say about a woman? There are people who will tell you it says "damaged goods," "ugly," "distorted," "abnormal." I don't see it that way. To me, a missing breast says "Here is a woman who is lucky," because she detected her breast cancer early enough to treat it. It says, "Here is a woman who is sensible and decisive," because she dealt with her problem quickly and effectively. It says, "Here is a woman with self-respect, strength, and resilience," who has gone through a tough time and come back to her normal life as ready as ever to give and to receive love. It says, "You're going to like this woman."

Now, I know all those positive attributes are more or less invisible, while a lopsided chest is right there for everyone to see. And I know that you can feel lucky and proud to have gotten through breast cancer and still be worried sick about being rejected for the mark it has left on your body. Rejection is, after all, the central issue here; let's admit that right now. When women talk about the effects of losing a breast, we are not really talking about beauty or sexuality; we are talking about the fear of rejection.

We all know how much rejection hurts, especially in romantic relationships. I can't imagine there is an adult man or woman who has not felt that pain at least once, or who wants to feel it again. Rejection hurts deeply; it makes you feel that there is something wrong with you. It makes you feel like less of a person. Rejection is something we all fear; too often our fear of it is the very thing that brings it on.

A woman who believes that because she has had a mastectomy there is something wrong with her, that she is less of a person, not only expects rejection, she creates it. Rather than waiting to see if someone else will be turned off by her altered body, she declares herself unattractive and unworthy of love, then turns her own brutal judgment into reality by radiating tension and despair, and withdrawing emotionally from anyone who threatens to show her affection.

I think the worst mistake a woman can make after mastectomy is to withdraw from sex. A good sexual relationship is a major source of warmth and tenderness as well as excitement and pleasure, all of which can contribute to your healing and help you regain balance and a sense of well-being.

Life Goes On, or Gets Better

❍

A woman who has had a mastectomy is not any more likely to be rejected by her lover than anyone else is. Every intimate relationship involves risks. You take a chance every time you reveal a new aspect of yourself to someone, physically or emotionally, whether that someone is a new acquaintance or a long-time lover. It's scary, because the thought of being rejected, for any reason, is scary. But worrying about how a lover is going to react to a missing breast is a waste of energy. A missing breast doesn't mean anything to most men. They are far more likely to be turned off by your self-consciousness or your negative attitude toward yourself.

In 1979, photographers Daphna Ayalah and Isaac Weinstock produced an intriguing book of photographs and interviews called *Breasts*. One of the many women interviewed about their attitudes toward their breasts was a British anthropologist named Elizabeth, who had a mastectomy back when the operation was far more extensive and disfiguring than it is today. A divorced woman in her thirties, she dated a lot of men. "Because of the mastectomy," she said, "I always cut myself off from emotion slightly when I meet a man until I know how he is going to react. I just casually in conversation bring up the fact that I had breast cancer — 'I had a breast removed.' If they are frightened, they have the option to veer off. It's very interesting because it has never made anybody shy away....If anything, it's caused men to love me more and with more tenderness because they feel that I have suffered, and that has been a revelation to me. It's even given me *more* self-confidence, because if a man can feel that way about me...well, he is obviously not just relating to me for my beautiful body, so I must be some special person." [92]

Like Roberta Altman, like me — like most women with mastectomies, I imagine — Elizabeth worried that she would be rejected, then found that the problem existed only in her own mind. I cannot speak for women with reconstructed breasts. I think many of them do have problems because their artificial breasts do not look or feel natural. A nicely healed, flat chest, on the other hand, is not a problem at all. It doesn't interfere with movement or call attention to itself. At worst, it is neutral, neither offensive nor erogenous. At best, it is a graceful, interesting contour that makes your body different from millions of others. What really makes many women with mastectomies different, and desirable sex partners, however, has nothing to do with the physical shape of their bodies. It is their exuberance, their conscious joy in being alive. Both my husband and I feel that our sex life has improved since my mastectomy, and that its new level of excitement stems from the delight we both feel, every time, that we are both alive and still together to enjoy it.

Women who undergo radiation treatments or chemotherapy before or after mastectomy obviously have more to recover from than women like me who have surgery alone. If such treatments drain your energy and cause a lot of discomfort, you may want to put your sex life on hold for a while. Once the treatments are over, your vitality should return, and with it a renewed interest in sex.

It's the Relationship That's Important

If you're married or in a long-term relationship, your sex life probably won't change at all after mastectomy. You know each other well. He knows you've had breast cancer. If you're a bit sore or shy at first, expect him to be understanding and patient, for a *little* while. (It's your job to get over any initial sensitivity as quickly as you can.) If there is a change, it is likely to be for the better. An ordeal like mastectomy seems to bring out the gentleness in men, which makes them even better lovers. What's more, their increased gentleness and sensitivity usually continue long after the cancer experience has faded, because both partners find in it a new level of mutual appreciation and satisfaction.

If you're single and dating new people, you will undoubtedly feel some self-consciousness about your missing breast at first, and it may keep you from jumping quickly into sexual involvement, which is good. Spur-of-the-moment coupling and one-night stands are physically dangerous in this age of deadly sexual diseases and have always been emotionally risky. One of the positive effects of mastectomy is that it takes some of the urgency and impersonalness out of sex. It makes you want to have a good sense of a man, to trust him, before you reveal yourself to him, which increases your chances of developing a real and satisfying relationship, based on more than a needy moment or a physical attraction. When you do begin a sexual relationship, you'll know that he's interested in you, not your breasts.

Appearance is so overemphasized in our culture, we sometimes forget that it is not the most important thing about people. It certainly isn't what holds a relationship together, and it's not even what makes a sexual encounter satisfying. As my husband commented one day, "If appearance were what it's all about, people wouldn't be able to make love in the dark."

His comment got me thinking. Why *do* so many of us prefer to make love in the dark? I don't think it's because we're shy. I think it's because we instinctively know that our sense of sight, which dominates most aspects of our lives, actually fetters and distracts us during sex. We have to turn it off in order to let our far more intense and sexually exciting senses carry us away.

What's Really Sexy?

Think about what really excites you during sex. For me, and I suspect for most people, the sense of touch is strongest. If it isn't dark, I close my eyes to let my sense of touch take over. My whole body becomes extremely sensitive when I can't see, and gentle fingertips moving over my skin give me exquisite pleasure. I become more aware of the warmth of my lover's body close to mine, and it elicits a deep, erotic response. Other senses besides touch participate in sex as well. I know I am very sensitive to sound, especially the sound of my partner's voice. A deep male voice, soft and gentle, is very exciting to me, and I absolutely love the way some men's voices get huskier when they're sexually aroused. I'm also turned on by aromas—not perfumes or after-shave, but a man's natural smell. I can often tell from the way my husband's body smells that he is in the mood for sex. The aroma is subtle, but it's different from his usual smell, and it affects me immediately.

Hearing, smell, touch, and for many people, taste—these are the senses that excite us during sex, far more than sight. Of all of them, only touch has anything to do with your breast, and even a woman who has no breasts at all has a lot of very erotic places to be touched. "Your body is ninety-five percent the same," my husband said one day, "and I don't miss the five percent that's gone." The comment was more a declaration of his love than an objective calculation of the change in my body, which is why I cherish it.

Love has a way of amplifying all of our senses, as well as stoking our appetites, which makes it *the* major ingredient of good sex. If you have love in your relationship, it simply doesn't matter how many breasts you have. Love, however, doesn't do well in a hostile climate. The loss of a breast cannot change love, but your response to that loss, if it is negative enough, can. If you have negative feelings about your body, you will set a negative tone that your partner will sense. Lying beside you in bed, he will feel your discomfort and your fear, and it will make him uncomfortable and afraid to approach you. Men sometimes withdraw from their partners after mastectomy not because they aren't attracted anymore, but because they are afraid to hurt or offend. The space that grows between two people who stop touching each other and stop communicating can get very cold, and love doesn't thrive in the cold.

Your lover is going to look to you for a signal that it is all right to go on loving you, physically as well as emotionally. It's up to you to reassure him that you are not fragile or damaged. You have to show him you are strong and vigorous, that you are able and ready to feel and to give pleasure. Before you can convince him, you have to believe it yourself.

If you believe that because of your missing breast you are no longer "whole" or sexually attractive, you probably aren't going to have any more sex. Now, that may be all right with you. Lots of women live without sex. I did for years when I was younger. I didn't feel deprived, either, because there was no one in my life I wanted to be with. It's an advantage women have over men. We can live very nicely without sex at certain times in our lives. Men have a harder time because their sex drive is more persistent and less discriminating. If you really want to forego sex, you'll probably find it fairly easy to do. If, on the other hand, you want to be sexually active, in the same way you were before breast cancer or in a different way, you can do that.

Getting Going Again

If you want to continue as a sexually active woman, the thing you need most is a positive attitude. The prosthesis, the breast reconstruction, the carefully selected clothes—all those things people tell you that you need—none of them really makes any difference. What matters is you. If, deep inside, you feel sorry for yourself for having had breast cancer, if you think you are no longer a desirable woman, your feelings of anger or despair will show through everything you say and do, and will put people off. If, on the other hand, you feel fortunate to have come through your ordeal in good shape, regardless of the number of breasts you have left, and you are looking forward to many more years as the same loving and lovable person you have always been, then your optimism and good cheer will draw people to you.

To a surprising degree, how you see yourself determines how others see you. If you are comfortable with yourself, other people tend to feel comfortable around you. If you feel beautiful, you carry yourself as if you were beautiful, you act beautiful, and you are beautiful. Beauty is not as narrowly defined as we have been led to believe, nor is sexiness.

We all know people, male and female, who are not particularly good-looking but are very attractive. It is not the contours of their faces, or of their bodies, that draw you to them. It is something in the way they smile, the way they look at you, the way they stand, and move. There is some light burning inside that shines out through their eyes. They are people you want to be around. You can tell right away that they like themselves and that makes you feel that you are going to like them too.

What people see when they look at you is largely a function of what you put forth for them to see. If you focus your attention on your missing breast, others will focus on it too. If you accept your lost breast as a small change in your body and focus instead on yourself as a complete person, you will be surprised at how many people don't notice the change, and how many of those who know about it simply forget. I have had friends stop in the midst of a conversation when I made a reference to my cancer, and say, "I'd completely forgotten you had that."

The British anthropologist who talked about her mastectomy in the photo book *Breasts* found, to her amazement, that some of the women at her health club didn't even notice her breast was missing, although she regularly walked around the locker room naked. She marveled, "A couple of women with whom I have become friendly there have said to me that initially they didn't notice—standing right in front of me and talking to me—that I have a mastectomy! It's true because another time I mentioned it to a woman there and she looked at me in shock and exclaimed, 'My God, I never noticed!'" [93]

The key to having people accept you as normal and attractive after your mastectomy is in accepting yourself as normal and attractive. For some women that takes more time than for others. You shouldn't rush back into a sexual relationship or go out looking for a new one before you're ready. Sex is as individual and intensely personal as it is universal. Everyone must come to it on her own terms and in her own time. On the other hand, if you decide to take your time, don't wait too long; too much delay can make it harder to take the first steps back.

If you feel too self-conscious to enter, or reenter, a sexual relationship right away, start by doing something to get back on good terms with your body. Treat yourself to some nonsexual activities that are sensuous and physically relaxing. A bubble bath may be a good place to begin. Or a massage. You might buy yourself a bottle of perfume or body oil with an aroma you find arousing. Do your nails. Buy yourself some sexy underwear. Get a new hairstyle. Anything that makes you feel good about your body will begin moving you back toward an active sex life.

When you are ready to be with a partner, don't just leave everything to chance. Plan to be together someplace where you know you can feel comfortable and relaxed. If your first encounter is going to be at your place, indulge in a little stage setting to insure that you'll be able to get in the appropriate mood. I can't tell you what will work for you, but I don't have to. You know what makes you feel sexy. For myself, I would have a fire in the fireplace and a bottle of wine at the ready. I would rent a romantic movie or have some favorite music to dance to. You don't have to worry about what he will find romantic. You're the one who's making a comeback; surround yourself with whatever establishes the right mood for you.

If you don't feel completely confident the first time out, let him seduce you. Let him see that you want him, but that you're a bit shy. Most men will respond to a little encouragement and take the situation in hand. A man who is mature and sensitive and cares for you, will be supportive and will know enough to move slowly. You can just close your eyes and think about how good it feels to be wanted. Let him touch you. Let him undress you. Let him caress you and hold you and talk softly to you. You'll soon know for certain that all the necessary parts of you are still there, still responsive, and still capable of giving you great pleasure.

After the first time, it gets easier and it gets better. Many women discover that after breast cancer they have much deeper and more satisfying romantic relationships than ever before. My relationship with my husband certainly grew. I think it's because I found so many new parts of myself during my cancer ordeal—reservoirs of strength and insight that I hadn't tapped into before. Having experienced more of myself, I felt I had more to give, and at the same time I wanted to reach for more of Jay. There's also the new respect, and affection, I have for my body for having gotten me through a serious health crisis. And there's the new respect Jay has for himself, having passed some kind of internal character test by loving me just the same after I lost a breast as he did before. To be honest, though, when we're in bed together I don't think about why things are so good between us. I just close my eyes and enjoy it.

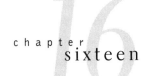

sixteen

When Your Cancer Crisis Is Over, Move On

Wisdom and strength are aftereffects of breast cancer.

The summer I was 10 years old I went to sleep-away camp for the first time. On the second day I came down with the mumps. They put me in the infirmary, which was presided over by a huge, silent black woman whose name I never learned. I was terrified of her. Nobody was allowed to visit me. A doctor came and gave me pills, but I didn't know how to swallow them, so I surreptitiously flushed them down the toilet. I sat alone in my bare little room feeling sorry for myself and writing heartbreaking letters to every relative and family friend in my address book. To my amazement, gifts started pouring in. Comic books, coloring books, puzzles—it was a bonanza. I felt powerful for the first time in my life. I wrote even more pitiful letters, for which I was lavishly rewarded....

I had decidedly mixed feelings the day the doctor released me. Although I was thrilled to be free again, I knew that during my absence the other girls had formed friendships and alliances, which are very important when you're 10 years old and in a strange new place. They were also somewhat wary of me because they knew mumps to be an extremely unpleasant and very contagious disease. I was made to leave my booty behind in the infirmary, no doubt, to be destroyed, so I ventured forth with nothing to offer but tales of my confinement and a budding sense of my own power.

Since I was the first person ever to be kept in the infirmary (it was the camp's first season as well as mine), everyone wanted to know what it was like. I regaled my bunkmates with stories of the letters I'd written and their amazing effect on softhearted adults. I vividly described flushing the pills down the toilet and the ominous sound of the nurse's heavy arm slapping against her side whenever she shook the thermometer down. Instead of the tale of misery they were expecting, I gave them an adventure story. I was accepted gladly back into the group and in a day or two my illness was forgotten in an exhilarating rush of swimming lessons, kickball games, and rowdy songs sung in the mess hall.

In some ways, coping with breast cancer made me feel like a child again, stuck in the infirmary with the mumps. Despite all the support and care I was getting, I often felt isolated and frightened. I resented my illness interfering with my life, and desperately wanted to be back among the healthy people I knew were enjoying themselves just outside. As soon as my ordeal was over, I hurried to rejoin the healthy world. Like my younger self at camp, I found greater joy in every activity because I had been kept from it for a time.

I was amazed at how easy it was to bounce back. Physically, breast cancer surgery doesn't leave you with a lot of handicaps. You get up one morning and realize you're feeling fine. You haven't lost a limb or had a vital organ weakened; you're not wearing a bag or adult diapers or laboring to breathe. Unless you have unusual complications, you can get right back into the swing of things, so long as you don't sabotage yourself, or allow others to sabotage you.

If you decide, as I did not, to undergo postsurgical treatment, such as radiation or chemotherapy, it will obviously prolong your medical ordeal. But eventually it too will be over, and you will be ready to return to your normal life. At that point you will have to decide if you are going to carry your cancer with you emotionally or if you are going to take what positive things you can from your experience and move forward.

Breast Cancer Hangover

Unfortunately, many women who are physically well again after breast cancer let their memories of being sick and their fears of a future recur-

rence keep them from rejoining groups and activities that would wel-
come them back. They dwell on their cancer experience instead of
leaving it behind. They let it put limits on the rest of their lives.

I think one thing that keeps some women focused on their cancer
is the overly cautious attitude of doctors who, trying to avoid giving
patients a false sense of security, instead burden them with lifelong
fears. The fact that your doctor won't say you're cured doesn't mean
your cancer is going to come back. Most women don't have recurrences of breast cancer. This is one instance where you have to understand your doctor's position and put his statements in context.
Although all your tests may show you to be cancer-free, he has no way
to tell for certain whether your cancer is gone for good. If he tells you
he thinks you're all right and then your cancer returns, or metastasizes,
he's afraid you'll feel you've been misled, and may even sue him. [94] So
the best most patients can expect from their doctors is a recitation of
the statistical odds. Dr. S. told me there was a 70 percent chance my
cancer would not return. I accepted those odds as definitely in my
favor and chose to be optimistic and return to my normal, active life.
A 70 percent chance of being cured may not sound very comforting to
you, but I found it a whole lot more reassuring than the 100 percent
chance that I'd be miserable every day if I chose to be pessimistic about
my future.

I refuse to live the rest of my life under a cloud. I hate the destructive and unnecessary "survivor" mentality that permeates our public
attitude toward breast cancer. Why do the media and cancer doctors
and researchers have to label every woman who does not die of breast
cancer a "survivor"? It marks us all in some vague way as walking
wounded and works to tie us forever, in our own minds, to an illness
that most of us experienced for only a few months. I never refer to
myself as a cancer survivor, and I encourage you to resist the label too.
There are far better ways to define yourself.

I am not suggesting that you try to forget your breast cancer experience—how could you?—but rather that you keep it in perspective, and recognize that virtually every major life experience, including the most trying, has potential for both good and bad results. What you make of it is up to you.

Twists of Fate

As apparently "bad" situations go, breast cancer is a doozie, but that doesn't mean it has nothing good to offer. It is the hard times, not the easy ones, that push us to grow. One of the reasons I find life endlessly fascinating is that you never know where an experience is leading you until you get there. Events that disrupt your life and force you to take an unexpected turn sometimes prove to be very good things in the end.

Many times in my life seeming disasters have turned out to be blessings in disguise. In 1981, I was suddenly evicted from the rent-controlled apartment I had lived in for nine years and had expected to live in forever. I was freelancing at the time, living alone, and making very little money. I searched in vain for another apartment I could afford. Finally, getting frantic, I rented a house well beyond my price range and began advertising for a roommate to split the cost. To my relief, I found one fairly quickly, but shortly before we were to move in, she changed her mind. I felt like my whole world was collapsing as I wrote a new roommate-wanted ad and posted it on a community bulletin board. It drew just one response—from a man. He was obviously a nice person, but I was sure I'd be more comfortable with a woman. It soon became obvious that it was him or no one, so, with considerable trepidation, I agreed to share the house with him—and that is how I met my husband.

It was a year and a half before we decided we were interested in each other, but in the spring of 1983 we were definitely in love. By then I had taken a full-time job and, despite the fact that neither of us was really happy at work, life was feeling awfully good. Too good, I guess. Within a few weeks of each other, we were both fired.

There we were, suddenly unemployed, with an expensive house, very little money in the bank, and no obvious prospects. I was upset and worried, but I also kept looking at Jay and thinking, we're together and we don't have to go to work tomorrow. One day my optimism got the better of me. We were driving back from the lighthouse at Pt. Reyes, where we had gone to look for migrating whales, when I took the leap.

"What would you think," I asked, "of putting all of our stuff in storage and going to Europe?" I held my breath.

"Sure," he said. So we gave up the house we could no longer afford, traded our meager savings for travelers' checks, and set off for two months of mostly unplanned, shoestring travel through Greece and Italy. It was the best two months of our lives.

If I hadn't been evicted, I never would have met Jay. If we hadn't both been fired, we wouldn't have taken the fantastic trip that cemented our relationship. If I hadn't had breast cancer, I would probably be editing someone else's book right now instead of writing my own.

I would never say that I am glad I had breast cancer. But I can't honestly say I am sorry either. For some women, breast cancer leads to prolonged illness and death. For me, it led to a resurgence of enthusiasm for life and a determination to become the person I had all but given up on ever being. My point is that you simply don't know how it's going to go for you. Why assume you're one of the unlucky ones and let sadness and despair rule your life? Chances are far better that you're one of the lucky ones—remember, the odds are in your favor, especially if you have found your cancer early.

Even when their treatment has apparently been successful, some women come out of their breast cancer ordeal carrying a heavy burden of anger, self-pity, fear, or shame. Where can such negativity possibly lead? Optimism is a far better attitude to take with you as you return to a healthy life. Besides making your steps lighter as you plug along, it will keep you looking for the best in whatever's ahead.

It's Up to You to Set the Tone

As you reclaim your place in the healthy world, you may find that you have to discourage family and friends from pitying you at first. After all, we have all been conditioned to think of women with breast cancer as weakened and depressed. Surprise those around you with your good humor and confidence. Show them that you're okay again and don't need to be tiptoed around or feared. If you give them the right cues, most will be happy, and relieved, to respond to you in a positive way.

You really can't fake good feelings, though, not with close friends and family members. They'll see right through a "brave" act and be confused and even more worried about doing and saying the right thing. So don't pretend you feel good about yourself if you don't. Instead, work on getting to a place where you really do feel glad to be alive and healthy again and are enthusiastic about the future. Then let those good feelings show.

Some women feel self-conscious after breast cancer and so avoid new relationships. If you do that, you'll be depriving yourself and all your future friends not only of the good times you could have together, but also of the wisdom and strength you have gained through your experience. Having been through a major life crisis, you have much to offer. You are not "damaged goods," but someone who has felt the fragility of life and understands the foolishness of wasting it. Regardless of your age, you are now an elder among the females of our tribe, someone who carries a special knowledge that deserves to be honored and shared.

Rather than letting uneasy feelings about your body hold you back, get out and make new friends, especially women friends. Talk freely with any of them who want to hear about your cancer experience. Your insights will encourage them; your joy in being alive will inspire them; your knowledge will help them overcome their ignorance and take better care of themselves. Because of your friendship, they will be more careful and less afraid.

I am convinced that American women would be less frightened of breast cancer if they talked more with women who have had it. As things are now, most women get their information from television, newspapers, magazine stories, and books that almost always focus on the minority of women with breast cancer who die of it, ignoring the many more who go on to live full and healthy lives. The Breast Cancer Research Foundation reported in October 1997 that 65 percent of women they surveyed wrongly believed that breast cancer is the leading killer of women today. Sixty-nine percent overestimated their risk of getting the disease. [95] A month later, a survey by the National Council on the Aging revealed that older women fear breast cancer more than other diseases they are far more likely to die of. Researcher Vincent T. Covello observed, "The focus groups support the findings that much of women's concerns about breast cancer, in particular, come from extensive media coverage on the topic." [96] And lack of someone experienced to talk to about it, I would add. Just by sharing what we've learned, you and I can begin to correct the misconceptions.

When you advise other women not to worry excessively about getting breast cancer, remember to caution yourself not to worry excessively about yours returning. Some women are so focused on that possibility, they imagine every new ache or pain is a sign that their cancer is recurring. Their constant vigilance and frequent panic-stricken visits to the doctor sap their energy and drain the joy from their (and their loved ones') lives nearly as much as a relapse would. Don't let what might happen tomorrow or next year ruin your good time today. If your cancer returns, you will know it soon enough; you don't need to drive yourself crazy watching for it.

Be a Better You

Even if they're not preoccupied with the possibility of a recurrence, some women have trouble returning wholeheartedly to their previous lifestyle because they are depressed by the thought that they are not the same as they were before. It is true. Breast cancer changes a woman, physically, psychologically, and emotionally. If you try to pretend you are the same, you are going to suffer from all sorts of internal and external conflicts. I think this is one reason breast reconstruction bothers me so much. It encourages women to pretend that by removing physical evidence of the disease, you can wipe out its psychological effects. You cannot.

The rush, on the part of both patients and doctors, to counteract the psychological and emotional effects of breast cancer assumes that those effects are negative. The fact is, however, that for many women they are not negative at all. Discovering that you have the strength to cope with a major life crisis without falling apart is quite positive. Learning that your value as a person has more to do with your patience, honesty, determination, wisdom, and love than with the size, or number, of your breasts is very positive. Realizing that you have something of value to contribute to the people in your life and your community, and perhaps beyond, is extremely positive, and energizing besides.

The reason breast cancer packs such a wallop psychologically and emotionally is that it demands that you grow up, which, though it can be painful, is ultimately a good thing. Breast cancer demands that you come to terms with your body as it really is (something women normally try to avoid) and reexamine the cultural myths that have shaped your attitudes in the past. For those who are willing to accept the challenge, a new kind of peace that is rooted in self-understanding and self-acceptance is the reward.

My own breast cancer experience made me see for the first time how completely my mind, body, and emotions are interconnected, how a blow to one immediately affects the others. In the beginning, as I made the decisions and selected the treatments that would change the contours of my body, I tended, as I imagine most women do, to measure my options and my self-image against the popular, mostly physical definitions of womanhood. But I soon found myself tangling with a much more complicated definition of myself as a human being. I discovered it is a short step from "Who will I be without my breast?" to "Who am I?"

Some women refuse to deal with the deeper questions that inevitably arise, perhaps because they are afraid of the answers. I have heard of women who as long as five years after a mastectomy still cannot bring themselves to look at their scar, or let their husbands look at it. These are surely women who went into surgery without first untangling the web of emotion that bound their breast and ego together, so that the scalpel that removed the one could not avoid doing extensive damage to the other.

Don't be afraid to look into yourself. You may, as I did, discover fortitude and insight you never knew you had. If you come across negative attitudes that are keeping you from functioning at your best, you'll still come out ahead. The darkest shadows vanish when a light is trained on them, and people who confront their weaknesses often find inspiration to change. There is a special kind of strength that comes from facing yourself, a strength that has sustained many women as they coped with the challenges of breast cancer. I have felt that strength in myself and in others.

Several months ago I went to a panel discussion at my HMO on life after breast cancer. The majority of both the panel and the audience were former breast cancer patients. I went expecting an atmosphere heavy with self-pity and desperation. Instead I found myself surrounded by level-headed, enthusiastic women anxious to share their insights and their coping tricks. It was one of the most positive meetings I have ever attended. None of the hundred-plus women there looked particularly sick or sounded depressed.

I looked around the room and wondered, where are the doctors? Why aren't they here to listen to these bright, energetic women? Every doctor who treats women with breast cancer should be required to attend a meeting like that. They would certainly learn some useful things, and perhaps seeing so many women thriving after breast cancer would get them to lighten up a bit. The pessimistic medical view of life after breast cancer drags women's spirits down. If your doctor implies that you're going to have a tough time getting on with your full and happy life, look him in the eye and tell him, for all of us, that you're going to do just fine.

What Lies Ahead?

When you've finished your treatment, be sure you step out into the world looking ahead, not back. Marvelous opportunities await you.

Even while you're still in treatment, I think it's a good idea to begin thinking about what you're going to do in your after-cancer life. The excitement of it will brighten, and perhaps even shorten, your recovery time. Perhaps there are ways you can make your current job more interesting and more fulfilling. Perhaps it's time for a new job. Or perhaps your aspirations have to do with a hobby, a sport, or volunteer work in your church or community. Think again about all the things you've wanted to do but never got around to, and start putting together plans to do some of them at last. Imagine how you will feel functioning at the highest creative level you are capable of. Don't be afraid to dream; dreams are what keep the spirit alive and the wheels of the mind turning.

As you sketch out your plans, don't worry about being too old or having been through too much to start new projects, or even a new career. Plenty of people have blossomed anew late in their lives, even without the advantage of the new vigor that comes with returning to health after a serious illness. James Michener, for instance, was 40 when his first novel was published. Are you well past 40? Most breast cancer patients are. Then, how about Grandma Moses? She began painting in her 80s. Golda Meir, having raised a family and had a long career as a teacher, became Prime Minister of Israel at 71.

It's not necessary to have a role model, but I think it helps to have someone you admire and want to emulate. As you look into the field that attracts you, you will undoubtedly find people whose accomplishments are inspiring. If you pick someone you know, you can talk to that person and perhaps gain her support and advice. If your role model is someone famous and beyond your reach, as mine is, stick a picture up on the wall to inspire you.

Don't limit yourself by thinking you have to do what others like you have done. Maybe no woman, or no one with a background similar to yours, has accomplished what you dream of doing. That's okay. You can be the first. Don't worry about setting your sights too high, either. Maybe you won't get all the way to your goal. So what? You will have a fine time trying, and you will certainly have some wonderful experiences along the way. What's more, with your heart and mind focused on your grand scheme, you won't have time to think about the limitations breast cancer is supposed to have imposed on you (what are they again?). It's hard to feel diminished when you're expanding in so many ways every day.

Whether your goals relate to women's health issues or not, the vigor and enthusiasm with which you pursue them can help to change the way women with breast cancer are seen by the public. You don't need to announce the fact that you've had breast cancer, but please don't hide it either. Everyone should know that each year thousands of women come back from an episode of breast cancer to enjoy their lives and contribute to their families, jobs, and communities even more than they did before they became ill.

Time and again I have seen a look of amazement on the faces of acquaintances and colleagues when I tell them I've had a mastectomy. At first they find it hard to reconcile their image of the sad, depleted cancer victim with my obvious good health and high spirits. They often comment that my recovery is exceptional, but I refuse to let them get away with that. When I was younger I ran into my share of narrow-minded folks who told me, "You're Jewish, but you're not like the others. I like you." I would snap back (I was more explosive then) "I am like the others, damn it. It's your image that's all wrong." I'm more patient now, and I calmly explain to the misinformed that most women are just fine after breast cancer—as healthy and energetic and capable as anyone else out there.

I know I've shattered a few preconceptions, but it's going to take a lot more healthy, feisty post-breast-cancer women strutting their stuff to convince the world we're far from being the broken dolls they imagine us to be.

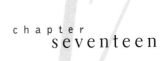
Losing a Breast, Finding a Voice

If you want things to change, you have to speak up.

In the last chapter I urged you to leave your cancer experience behind once your ordeal is over, and go on with your life. I think it is important to us as individuals to do so. At the same time, I think it is important to the women who will face breast cancer in the future (including, surely, many of our daughters) that we not walk away completely....

I'm not saying that we who have been through breast cancer owe something to those who will follow us. I don't believe in obligation, but I do believe in opportunity.

We are constantly being reminded that the number of women with breast cancer is very large and growing each year. We are told it is a tragedy, and surely it is, but it also has its positive side. Our increasing numbers mean greater power to demand and influence change. Millions of American women have had encounters with breast cancer. Each year about 180,000 more join our ranks. If just 1 percent of us were to join together and speak out, we would create a presence impossible to ignore. We could change the focus of discussion that has been dominated by politicians and medical professionals for too long.

Oh, I know there are a lot of breast cancer activists out there already, lobbying for more research dollars, better treatments, and more public education. I admire their efforts, but I think we need to reevaluate the direction in which they, and the prevailing images of breast cancer, are taking us.

It seems to me, looking at breast cancer from the vantage point of my own experience, that too much of the current fundraising, research, and available treatments are focused on the minority of patients with life-threatening, advanced cases, while the majority of us—those with early, treatable cancers—get little attention. I am as anxious as anyone to see treatments developed that will cure advanced breast cancer. But I am equally anxious for a way to identify and release from treatment those patients whose cancer is gone after their initial round of surgery.

As long as current attitudes remain entrenched, I fear that breast cancer research will continue to favor extreme, often dangerous, treatments that are, not coincidentally, very profitable for their manufacturers, and that those treatments will continue to be inflicted on patients who have already been cured. I fear that educational programs will continue to publicize exaggerated statistics that frighten women and keep some away from the exams that could catch their cancers early. And I fear that mastectomy patients will continue to be pressured into unnecessary cosmetic surgeries.

Standing Up, Standing Out

As a rule, we who have had breast cancer and returned to health do not see ourselves as a force for change, or even as a community. Instead of sharing our experiences and our newfound strength and wisdom, most of us rush to disguise our altered bodies, making ourselves invisible to the world at large and unrecognizable to each other. It is unfortunate, because women who have been through breast cancer are in a perfect position to lead the way toward a saner and healthier future for all women. In general we are older, more experienced, and bolder than the average woman. We're battle-scarred and worldly-wise, and we've confronted our feelings about our bodies in a way most women have not. I think we could begin to make things better just by becoming more available to one another.

I am not talking about signing up to be a Reach To Recovery or information center volunteer, although both are positive and helpful things to do. I am talking about something far more basic, something anyone can do even if you have no free time to offer. I'm talking about simply accepting yourself and letting other women see who you are.

Imagine for a moment what would happen if all of the women who have had a mastectomy stopped hiding the fact, and the sight of a one-breasted woman became common. Now, I don't wear a prosthesis, so it's pretty obvious to anyone who cares to notice that I am lopsided. Still, in the four years since my mastectomy, not a single person has come up to me to ask about it. If people became used to seeing one-breasted women on the street, would they lose their horror of it, and their fear of mentioning it? I can picture a woman I don't know approaching me.

"Excuse me," she might say, "but I noticed you're missing a breast. I found a lump in my breast last week and I'm terrified." "Oh," I might answer, "don't worry yourself sick. You know, I had two lumps in my breast, both malignant, and I'm fine. Have you been to a doctor?"

As quickly as that, the door would swing open and I would share what I'd learned with someone who desperately wanted to know. Perhaps later in the day she would sight another one-breasted woman and talk to her, too, and compare her experience with mine.

It would be such a small thing, but it could be the beginning of a whole new way women look at each other's bodies and their own.

Perhaps on another day a woman recovering from mastectomy would stop me and say, "I see you didn't have reconstruction. Is it hard living without your breast?" And I would chuckle and say "No, it's fine." And she would say, "What does your husband think?" And I would say, "He doesn't miss it at all." And perhaps one more woman would save herself the pain and cost and psychological assault of unnecessary cosmetic surgery.

I think that with thousands of healthy, energetic postmastectomy women casually sharing their stories, the frightening popular image of breast cancer would quickly change. It bothers me greatly that the very women we most need to hear from are the most silent. Many feel, I think, that they have nothing to share because their tumors were small and quickly taken care of. How wrong they are! As I talked with friends during and after my recovery, I realized that my breast cancer experience was important precisely because it was not dramatic or painful or particularly disruptive of my life. The very fact that it was not the expected horror story made it reassuring, and even inspiring. By keeping silent, we who have had relatively easy experiences have helped distort the truth about breast cancer and have allowed its doom-and-gloom image to go unchallenged, darkening hundreds of thousands of women's lives.

It is fair, and important, to ask what would happen to breast cancer research if the disease lost its terrifying image. Certainly, portraying breast cancer in the darkest possible terms has helped to keep research dollars flowing. I have serious doubts, however, as to how much good the current research approach is doing us.

It sometimes seems to me that our biggest problem is not that there is too little breast cancer research, but that too much of the research that is being done is pointless. I believe strongly that we should be spending our research time and dollars on trying to discover what causes the disease and finding more effective ways to treat it, not on guessing who might get it.

If it were up to me, all the programs now concentrating on risk-factor research would switch tomorrow to one of three more practical lines of inquiry. One group would devote its efforts to looking for a cure. Another would work at developing a conclusive test to confirm when cancer is gone, freeing a majority of women with early breast cancer from the scourge of unneeded, invasive treatments. The third group would look for the cause of the disease, which I suspect is to be found not in ourselves but in our poisoned environment. (If we could identify and eliminate an external cause, or group of causes, we could forget about developing "preventive" drugs.) I assume, I hope not naively, that these areas are already being vigorously explored. Perhaps with the added help of researchers and funding now being used to chase down risk factors, success would come sooner.

Politically Speaking

I have no illusions that my arguments will do much to change the way research is currently oriented. The status quo is ingrained and has powerful supporters. In 1998 I sent a letter to my U.S. Senator, Dianne Feinstein, who sponsored the bill to create a breast cancer stamp to raise more money for research. I laid out my concerns and asked that she carefully consider how the new funds would be spent. I guess she didn't have time to read my letter, because the form letter I got in return didn't address my points. I tried again, this time writing to an assistant in her office, identified in the form letter as the person in charge of listening to voters on the subject of breast cancer. He never responded at all.

I guess a couple of letters from one voter are pretty easy for a politician to ignore, even a female politician who claims breast cancer as an issue of great importance to her. But what if thousands of women wrote to dozens of senators and representatives? Do you think they would begin to take notice? I do.

If we made sure that all the funds currently available for breast cancer research were being used to find solutions that will actually help us, perhaps we wouldn't be so desperate for more funding—although I'd like to see that too.

While I think it's very important to get the policymakers on our side, I don't think we can afford to wait for them to act. Given the attitudes of our government at present, and the tremendous power big business has to influence its direction, I don't expect real change to come from above. We have to take responsibility for getting things moving; we have to make it clear that we are serious.

We women tend to think of ourselves as powerless to affect the political and commercial interests that control so much that happens in our lives. In fact, we are not powerless at all; we're just distracted and disorganized. Women are the majority in this country. We control a majority of the votes, and we spend a majority of the consumer dollars. If we ever made up our minds to do so, we could shake the politicians who decide on national priorities, and the big businesses that use us so shamelessly, right down to their roots.

Cast Your Vote at the Cash Register

I actually do believe that our lifestyle makes us more susceptible to breast cancer, and other diseases as well—just not in the way the risk-factor researchers suggest. I think we put ourselves in more danger through the products we select at the supermarket than through our decisions on when to have children or whether to breastfeed. I believe our poor eating habits and sedentary routines weaken our bodies, which then cannot fight off the effects of the poisons we unknowingly—and often unavoidably—eat, drink, handle, and breathe. Unlike the size of our bones or our age at the onset of menopause, these are lifestyle elements we can change. What's more, I believe there would be a tremendous bonus in changing the way we choose the products we buy; by cleaning up our personal habits, we would pressure many of the producers who are polluting our environment to clean up theirs.

If you doubt that there is a connection between rampant pollution and cancer, I suggest you read Sandra Steingraber's frightening book *Living Downstream*.[97] This carefully researched call to action by an ecologist who was struck by bladder cancer in her twenties makes it clear that the levels of dangerous chemicals in our air, water, and food are far higher than most of us suspect. Steingraber traces many of these contaminants to agricultural and industrial practices that have become commonplace since World War II, including an astronomical increase in the use of pesticides. As the volume of these chemicals has increased, so has the rate of cancer—all kinds of cancer. Many of the pesticides now in common use have been specifically linked to breast cancer.

The reason thousands of businesses are allowed to contaminate our world is a complicated mix of money, power, and politics. The reason we keep buying the products those businesses produce is … what? Ignorance? Laziness? Blind trust? Self-destructiveness? A belief that we have no power to bring about change, and therefore no choice?

I don't believe the battle against diseases like breast cancer can be won until we, as individuals and as a nation, take serious action against environmental pollution. Official progress has been too little and way too slow. While hundreds of thousands of us are diagnosed with cancer each year, scientists complain that it is difficult to definitely identify chemicals that cause disease, and economists worry about how businesses will suffer if we hold them to the lofty standard of not poisoning us. Well, I am neither a scientist nor an economist, but I know that if products stop selling, their manufacturers will either go out of business or switch to products that will sell. If, as a result of our more careful buying, businesses that are reckless with our safety go under, good riddance to them. I am ready for the new, more conscientious businesses that will spring up to take their place.

The good news is that becoming smarter consumers is much easier than you might think. The obvious, most basic place to start is with our food. Even those of us too busy to think about scientific studies and political maneuvering can see that eating pesticides is not good for our health. Most of the crops raised on American farms today, including many ingredients in all those processed "convenience" foods we are so fond of, are raised with chemical aids. Not all foods exposed to chemicals contain harmful residues, but given the lack of dependable public information, I don't know which ones are safe, and neither do you. On the other hand, there are foods we can buy that we are certain have not been chemically adulterated. In California, where I live, certified organic fruits and vegetables, dairy products, and even meats are available in many markets.[98] True, in most cases organically produced food costs more, but it doesn't cost as much as cancer. Besides, the rules of the marketplace are in our favor: the more organic food we buy, the more companies will turn to producing it, and before long, prices will fall.

If you're not already buying organic food, try this. The next time you shop, drop one highly processed or chemically sprayed item from your list and replace it with a fresh organic food. That's not too hard. The time after that, replace two. If your market doesn't carry organic foods, seek out the manager and ask when they're going to start. If enough of us persist, we should soon begin seeing significant changes. Our preference for chemical-free foods will give more farmers reason to clean up their farms. (Many say they would like to, if consumers would support them.) More organic products will be available in our stores at lower prices. A shrinking market for pesticide-treated foods should also result in a lower demand for pesticides, which should in turn start some chemical companies looking for safer products to make. Less manufacturing of poisons means less pollution and less on-the-job exposure for workers, all important steps in the right direction.

Poisonous Habits

Many of us have been unaware that we are eating pesticide residues on food, but we knowingly bring other poisons into our homes, either not thinking about the danger or thinking we have no choice. When my daughter Rebecca was in first grade, she came home from school with head lice. Like most parents, I panicked at the sight of those horrible bugs crawling in her hair and, not knowing what else to do, I applied the bug killer sold for the purpose of removing them. With second grade came more lice, and more pesticide on her head. In third grade, she came home with lice that were resistant to the poison I'd been using;[99] they were just as hardy after the application as before. Our pediatrician said there was a stronger pesticide available by prescription, but it was so toxic she didn't want to use it.

Jay was determined to find a safe alternative. He went to an herb shop and came back with three little bottles of natural oils—eucalyptus, rosemary, and pennyroyal. A book he'd found said those oils, mixed into olive oil, would kill the lice and keep them from coming back. I was skeptical, but I mixed the concoction, combed it through Rebecca's hair, and left it overnight as instructed. In the morning I washed it out and looked for lice. They were gone.

Since that incident, Jay and I have found other ways to avoid using poisons in our home. He read somewhere that Vaseline smeared around a hole where ants come into the house will form a barrier to keep them out. We tried it on the plastic plate of an electrical outlet that had become an ant highway from the back yard to our kitchen counter. It worked great. The only drawback was that we had to keep wiping away the carcasses of ants that got stuck in the goop. I'd rather do that than have poison on my kitchen counter.

We've never used weed killers in the garden, but many, many people do. According to Sandra Steingraber's research, weed killers are among the most widely used poisons in the country, and among the most dangerous. I pull weeds by hand in our yard. We don't have very many anyway because we dug up the lawn years ago and planted flowering trees and bushes instead. We did it because lawns don't make much sense in drought-prone California. Maybe, given the carcinogenic nature of weed killers, they don't make sense anywhere else either. Perfect green, trimmed lawns are just one more example of our American obsession with unnatural beauty, for which we are recklessly endangering our health.

Let's Change the World

Eliminating a few dangerous chemicals from my home hasn't made a lot of difference in the world. But if you do the same, we will have twice the impact. If millions of us did it, the effect would be revolutionary.

To really clean up our environment, of course, we will have to swear off more than just weed killers and pesticides. Other products we use regularly are every bit as dangerous. The chemicals used in dry cleaning, for instance, have been identified as particularly carcinogenic. I have tried for years to buy only washable clothes simply because dry cleaning is so expensive. Now I think about what would happen if large numbers of women stopped taking our clothes to the dry cleaner and refused to buy "dry clean only" clothes until the process was made safe. I suspect dry cleaners would start looking for new ways to clean delicate fabrics. (I understand there is a promising nontoxic "wet-cleaning" process already being offered in a few locations.) Clothing manufacturers would have to switch to washable fabrics or close up shop. Under such consumer pressure, you can bet a new, safe cleaning process would soon be widely available. Then dangerous dry-cleaning chemicals could be banned, and we could pull out our wools and silks and rayons again, proud of what we've accomplished.

Using the same approach, health-conscious consumers could pressure the industries that produce polluting detergents, dyes, and solvents to find nontoxic alternatives. We might even spur the long-overdue development of widely available solar and wind energy, gasoline-free cars, and a kazillion other safe and sane products.

I don't think I am overestimating the power we as consumers have to change the world we live in. We have already begun. The selective spending of a relatively small number of us has put organic produce in our supermarkets [100] and homeopathic remedies on the shelves of mainstream drugstores. By making simple changes in the way we deal with trash, we have made the recycling of paper, glass, and some plastics routine. By withholding our dollars, we convinced tuna fishermen to curb the brutal killing of dolphins. Now we need only increase our numbers and broaden our demands.

While we use our spending patterns to clean up the future, we can use our votes to clean up the past. Today, self-serving big businesses have the ear of many politicians; tomorrow our voices could drown them out. If we inform political candidates that we will vote only for representatives who will force those who have polluted our environment to clean it up, immediately and at their own expense, they will have to take notice. All the money sent their way by the big polluters won't do them any good if we cast our votes against them.

None of these actions in our defense and the defense of our loved ones would take much time or effort. None of them requires you to attend rallies or donate to political organizations. You and I can begin changing the world simply by changing our attitudes. If cancer, or fear of cancer, is part of your life, perhaps you should be doing a little something to help stop it.

Will You Still Love Me... (A Chapter for the Men)

We all need to rethink our attitudes toward women's breasts.

Breast cancer affects all of us, men as well as women. Our lives are intertwined. Men certainly know that if breast cancer strikes a woman they love, their lives will be changed by it too. What many men don't understand, I think, is that their attitudes affect the way women see their own bodies and influence the decisions women make about their health....

If you are reading this chapter, chances are that a woman you are close to has breast cancer now. Unfortunately, most of us, both women and men, don't learn much about the disease until we or someone close to us already has it. You have undoubtedly heard some scary things about breast cancer, so the first thing you should know is that most women who get it don't die of it. I hope if the woman you love has been diagnosed with breast cancer, she will be one of the more than 70 percent who undergo successful treatment and return to a healthy life. Her chance of doing so may depend on you.

When a woman is stricken with a potentially fatal disease, her mind should obviously be focused on doing whatever is necessary to stop that disease and regain her health. Women diagnosed with breast cancer, however, are often worried about something else. The woman you love may in fact be worried that if she loses a breast, as many women with breast cancer do, she will lose your love. This may sound incredible to you—of course you love her, not just her breasts—and yet there are women so sure that their partners will leave them if they have just one breast that they will not allow a breast to be removed.

These days most breast cancers are found early and can be successfully treated. But treatment almost always means surgery. If your partner refuses to undergo surgery for fear of losing you, her cancer will continue to grow and will probably kill her. If she accepts surgery but has a lumpectomy rather than a mastectomy, in order to keep her breast there for you, she will have to have follow-up radiation treatments, which can cause long-term health problems. Choosing a breast cancer treatment is one of the most important and difficult decisions of a woman's life, which is why you need to speak up.

Does the woman you love know how you feel about her? Does she believe that you will love her just as much with one breast as with two? Think carefully before you answer. There is, I think, a major misunderstanding between men and women on this question.

I have conducted my own informal survey among the men I know, both married and single. Every man I asked said he would not feel any differently toward the woman in his life if she lost a breast. He would still love her and still find her sexually attractive. Yet most women think men care tremendously about women's breasts. All the low-cut dresses and the padded and push-up bras attest to that, to say nothing of the booming business in cosmetic breast surgery. Do you think women put so much effort and money into enhancing their breasts to please themselves? Of course not. They do it to attract and please men—the very men who say they don't care all that much. Either the men I talked to were lying to me, or there is a huge, and dangerous, communication gap here.

I think most men don't really care that much about breasts. I think they did once, when they were teenagers, and their hormones were running wild, and the girls at school began developing breasts you could see pushing out under their shirts. I think then breasts were fascinating and exciting and fun. As adults, most men have found much more satisfying ways of relating to women. But our cultural obsession with breasts is still around—in jokes, magazines, movies, videos, calendars—and it's easy to get pulled in. I think most men don't mean any harm by going along with it, and I certainly don't think they realize that their innocent fun may be endangering the women they care most about.

You see, we women have taken men's focus on our breasts seriously. Many of us have come to believe that without good-looking breasts we'll never be noticed or loved. We have even accepted the idea that the bigger our breasts are, the better, which goes directly against our own perceptions and experience.

You may be surprised to hear that women with large breasts mostly hate them. I was surprised, as I talked to large-breasted women, to hear how much trouble their breasts have caused them. Since I don't have very large breasts, I hadn't ever thought much about it. One woman complained that the extra weight makes it impossible for her to run comfortably. Another talked about the deep ridges in her shoulders caused by her bra straps and the aching she feels in her back by the end of every day. A third recalled with obvious pain the teasing and taunting she endured as a teenager and the assumption on the part of the boys in her school that because she had big breasts she was both stupid and easy. To all of these women, and many more, large breasts are a problem, not a point of pride. So why do millions of women wish for bigger breasts, and why on earth have hundreds of thousands risked surgery to add a cup size or two? Because of men.

The real problem here is not that men want women to have big breasts and women feel they have to have them. The problem is a lack of communication. For some reason it's apparently easy for a man to tell a woman "I love your breasts," and very difficult for him to say "Your breasts are not important to me." Perhaps it's because men are as manipulated by the popular culture as women are. They think they're *supposed* to be all hung up on women's breasts, so they don't want to admit that they're not. Maybe you think your partner will be disappointed if you tell her that her breasts aren't as important to you as she thinks. Take it from me, if you tell her you love her and would even if she had no breasts at all, she won't be disappointed; she'll be delighted, and relieved.

It seems to me there are a lot of people these days trying to drive men and women apart. In the past few years a growing number of preachers and therapists, and even a poet or two, have been declaring that men and women should return to their traditional roles, meaning that women should go back to being silent and dominated by men. I doubt that all the chest-beating (and drum-beating) will convince many women to return to the subservient position we held and detested for so long, but I fear it may succeed in setting back the progress men and women have made toward being able to talk to each other.

I'm sure you will be there physically for your partner during her breast cancer crisis, available to drive her to medical appointments and do extra chores so she can rest. That's great, but she needs something more from you, something that requires real strength and maturity. She needs you to be available to her emotionally, ready and willing to listen and to talk about what both of you are really feeling. She needs to know that she can make the decisions that are best for her health without worrying that if her body changes you will turn away from her.

If you're a man whose life has not been touched by breast cancer, it's still important for you to let the woman you love know that her breasts are not the reason you are with her. No one knows why some women get breast cancer and others don't, or who is likely to be stricken, or when. We do know that it's important for every woman to check regularly for signs of trouble. In general, the serious breast cancer cases are those that are found too late, after the cancer has begun to spread to other parts of the body. If your partner believes that losing a breast would mean losing your love, she may refuse to have a mammogram or to do breast self-exams out of fear of finding a lump. By avoiding these simple precautions, she increases the chance that if breast cancer should strike, it would not be found in time to save her.

Finally, you should know that even in this era of high-tech medicine, most breast tumors are found by women themselves or by their lovers. Yes, their lovers. Many a man's sensitive touch has detected a tiny tumor and saved a woman's life. So don't think I am suggesting that a man shouldn't ever focus on a woman's breasts. Paying attention to her breasts, stroking and fondling them, is not only enjoyable for both of you, it could be a health advantage as well. It is a problem only when such physical intimacy replaces other forms of communication and becomes your only way of relating to her. Enjoy each other's bodies, but be sure she knows that she is far more to you than the sum of her physical parts.

Afterword

A phrase that has stuck with me since childhood is one I heard chanted many times in the synagogue: *Chazak, chazak, v'nishazaik,* "Be strong, be strong, and we shall strengthen one another." It comes to me now as I complete this book and look toward the future.

In 1999, four years after my breast cancer crisis, breast cancer is still a terrifying presence in many women's lives and an unsolved mystery to medical researchers. There may be little we, as individuals, can do to speed up the discovery of a cure, but there is a great deal we can do to counteract the terror.

The most important step we can take in that direction is also the simplest: we can start talking to each other. Openly. Honestly. About what we've learned and what we fear, about our hopes and our worries, our pain and our confusion. If there's one thing I know for certain about breast cancer, it's that when women share their knowledge and their strength, the fear begins to dissolve.

Our lives sometimes seem so different from each other's that it is hard to know where to look for common ground, especially when it comes to subjects we consider deeply personal. What do young women have in common with old? Single with married? Straight with gay? Professionals with homemakers? Too often, distracted by appearances, we look right past each other, never seeing that we are more similar than different. Strangely, breast cancer, the disease that has given us all something to fear, has also given us a meeting place and a reason to seek each other out.

If you want to strike an immediate blow against the emotional devastation of breast cancer, talk to other women, those who are close to you and those you happen to meet. Talk not only about cancer, but about self-image, yours and theirs, and the narrow ideas of female beauty we have all been pressured to accept. The feelings of connection that blossom in such conversations are comforting and invigorating. They not only boost the confidence of women who are coping with the stresses of illness, but show us all a way out of the ignorance and isolation that feeds our fears.

I hope, now that you know most women with breast cancer regain their health and many feel their lives are better after cancer than before, you will approach your own breast cancer crisis with optimism and involvement rather than fear and resignation. A positive attitude may not be enough to turn aside a serious health threat, but without it you will surely miss the opportunities that come with the struggle. Growth, insight, and greater self-awareness and self-respect are all common outcomes of serious illness, and they outlast the discomfort and upheaval most people suffer.

I wish you well on your journey, because breast cancer *is* a journey, and none of us knows at the outset where it will lead. To give yourself the best possible chance for success, be sure you take along your faith, your love of life, your sense of humor, and your curiosity, and choose for your companions on the road, both medical and personal, people who appreciate you for who you are and will help you not only to recover, but to flourish.

Notes

Chapter 1

[1] For a full-length study of the image of the female breast through history, see A History of the Breast by Marilyn Yalom (Knopf, 1997).

[2] In 1992, the FDA declared a moratorium on the use of silicone breast implants and called on manufacturers to document their safety. At the time it was estimated that between one and two million women in the United States had implants. According to the New York Times, about 430,000 women had filed claims against implant manufacturers. Legal actions mainly focused on Dow Corning, the largest. In 1993, the companies together offered to settle for $4.25 billion, of which Dow was to pay $2 billion. Instead, on May 15, 1995, Dow sought the protection of Chapter 11 bankruptcy. In February 1998, still in bankruptcy, Dow offered to pay $3 billion to 177,000 women over a period of 16 years. A story by the Associated Press on November 10, 1998, reported that Dow had submitted a $3.2 billion settlement proposal to the U.S. Bankruptcy Court. By then, more than 600,000 women had sued Dow. If the plan is approved, the report said, payouts could begin in the summer of 1999.

Chapter 2

[3] Figures such as this are always approximations and are usually expressed in round numbers. In March 1996, I attended a "Women's Health 2000" conference at the University of California, San Francisco (UCSF), which houses one of the country's most highly regarded breast cancer research centers. The medical experts who spoke there reported the annual U.S. breast cancer death rate as 45,000. Now it appears the number of deaths may be beginning to go down. The American Cancer Society has predicted 43,700 U.S. breast cancer deaths in 1999.

[4] Dr. Virginia L. Ernster, Ph.D., Vice Chair of the UCSF School of Medicine Department of Epidemiology and Biostatistics, was a featured speaker at the 1996 "Women's Health 2000" conference at UCSF. In the conference Resource Guide she listed the risk estimates for breast cancer quoted here and in the following paragraphs, which I have since seen confirmed in many publications.

[5] From the 1996 "Women's Health 2000" conference Resource Guide, op. cit., p. 8.

[6] These numbers for estimated risk are based on data used pretty consistently by medical authorities and reporters. I saw them first in the Resource Guide for the UCSF "Women's Health 2000" conference (op. cit.), and later in a number of books, including Roberta Altman's carefully researched *Waking Up, Fighting Back: The Politics of Breast Cancer* (Little, Brown, 1996). They were recently cited by Dr. Leslie Ford, associate director for early detection at the National Cancer Institute, in an interview in the January 31, 1999, *Parade* magazine.

[7] An article in January 1999 in the *New England Journal of Medicine* looked at breast cancer risk in 10-year spans and concluded, "the risk of breast cancer in any given decade of life never exceeds 1 in 34." (Phillips, Kelly-Anne, M.B., B.S., Gordon Glendon, M.Sc., and Julia A. Knight, Ph.D., "Putting the Risk of Breast Cancer in Perspective," *New England Journal of Medicine*, Volume 340, Number 2, January 14, 1999, p. 141.)

[8] According to Dr. Laura Esserman, Co-Director of the Breast Care Center at the UC San Francisco School of Medicine, 6 percent of women who get breast cancer have a family history of the disease. Estimates by other experts in the field vary slightly; all I have seen are between 5 and 10 percent. Two studies released in early 1998 demonstrated how rarely breast cancer is passed on through an inherited "breast cancer gene." In one study, conducted at the University of North Carolina and the University of Washington, 200 women with invasive breast cancer were tested for the gene. None of the black women (about half the subjects) carried the gene, and only 3.3 percent of the white women did. In the second study, conducted at the Fred Hutchinson Cancer Research Center in Seattle, 401 women with breast cancer were tested for the gene. Among those diagnosed before they were 35 years old, only 6.2 percent had the gene. Among those who were diagnosed before 45 and had close relatives

with breast cancer, only 7.2 percent had the gene. (Perlman, David, "Breast Cancer Test of Small Value," *San Francisco Chronicle*, March 25, 1998, p. A4.)

[9] Drs. Lila and Robert Nachtigall, in their book *What Every Woman Should Know: Staying Healthy After 40* (Warner, 1995, p. 137), write "[I]f you are an average American woman, only if you live to be 110 will your chances be one in nine."

[10] In the Resource Guide for the 1996 "Women's Health 2000" conference at UCSF (op. cit.), Dr. Virginia L. Ernster wrote: "[A]s many as 5–15% of women screened will have abnormal mammograms requiring additional procedures (including surgery) to determine whether breast cancer is present. But in the vast majority of these cases (around 95%) the abnormality is not breast cancer: these are referred to as 'false positives.'"

[11] Analysis of federal statistics, as reported in the February 1997 issue of the *University of California at Berkeley Wellness Letter*, revealed that from 1990 through 1995 deaths from breast cancer among American women declined by 6.3 percent. Although more than ten times as many women die of heart disease, in a survey conducted by the Breast Cancer Research Foundation in late 1997, some 65 percent of the women interviewed wrongly named breast cancer as the leading cause of death among women. ("U.S. Women Terrified of Breast Cancer," *San Francisco Chronicle*, October 4, 1997, p. A3.) In March 1998, officials at the Centers for Disease Control and Prevention in Atlanta and the National Cancer Institute reported that the rate of new lung cancers and lung cancer deaths among American women was rising, probably because more women are smoking. In January 1998, the American Heart Association reported that 505,440 American women died of cardiovascular diseases in 1995, the most recent year for which figures were available.

Chapter 3

[12] This new understanding of breast cancer cell growth was introduced in the 1970s. For a more detailed explanation, see *Dr. Susan Love's Breast Book*, second edition (Addison Wesley Longman/Perseus Books, 1995), p. 265. It is important to understand that numbers like these are always generalizations. Individual tumors may grow slower or faster.

[13] I am told that testing goes faster for many patients, especially those seeing private doctors. You may have a definite diagnosis in weeks, rather than the months it took me.

[14] According to "A Woman's Guide to Breast Cancer Diagnosis and Treatment," published in 1995 by the California Department of Health Services, eight out of ten breast lumps are harmless. (The state requires all California doctors to give the booklet to patients before biopsy or at the time of a diagnosis of breast cancer.)

[15] *Breast Cancer: The Psychological Effects of the Disease and Its Treatment* by Karin Gyllensköld, translated by Patricia Crampton (Tavistock Publications, 1982).

Chapter 5

[16] Runowicz, Carolyn D., M.D., and Donna Haupt, *To Be Alive: A Woman's Guide to a Full Life After Cancer* (Henry Holt and Company, 1995), p. 133.

[17] These two studies are discussed in *Remarkable Recovery: What Extraordinary Healings Tell Us About Getting Well and Staying Well* by Caryle Hirshberg and Marc Ian Barasch (Riverhead Books/G.P. Putnam's Sons, 1995), p. 216.

[18] Moyers, Bill, *Healing and the Mind* (Doubleday, 1993), p. 157.

Chapter 7

[19] In his best-selling book *Ageless Body, Timeless Mind* (Harmony Books, 1993, p. 20) Dr. Deepak Chopra writes about "a meticulous 1987 study from Yale" which showed that "breast cancer spread fastest among women who had repressed personalities, felt hopeless, and were unable to express anger, fear, and other negative emotions." People unable to express their strong emotions have long been referred to as having a "cancer personality." A number of other studies, including those by Dr. David Spiegel at Stanford, have shown that cancer patients who express their feelings fare better than those who do not.

[20] Steinem, Gloria, *Revolution from Within: A Book of Self-Esteem* (Little, Brown, 1992), p. 246.

Chapter 8

[21] I am indebted to Barbara Ehrenreich and Dierdre English and their excellent book *For Her Own Good: 150 Years of the Experts' Advice to Women* (Doubleday, 1978) for much of my understanding of the history and masculinization of the medical profession.

[22] Goodman, Ellen, *Value Judgments* (Farrar, Straus & Giroux, 1993), p. 61. Once I became aware of this phenomenon, I began noticing how widespread the practice of conducting all-male studies is. As I write this note, I am looking at a story in today's *San Francisco Chronicle* (March 5, 1999, p. A3), which reports on a major study on the connection between blood pressure and aging of the brain, conducted by the Alzheimer's Disease Center at the University of Kansas. All 414 subjects were men.

[23] A study by researchers at Harvard University and the University of Washington, published in the April 16, 1998, issue of *The New England Journal of Medicine*, concluded that women who have annual mammograms have a 50 percent chance of getting one false positive result within each 10 years. (See also [17] above.) According to the Medical Board of California's Action Report (October 1998, p. 8), "some studies show that mammography has an average false negative rate of 15%."

[24] Stabiner, Karen, *To Dance with the Devil: The New War on Breast Cancer: Politics, Power, and People* (Delacorte Press, 1997), p. 132.

[25] I have never found any explanation why, if estrogen is the cause of breast cancer, a woman's risk increases sharply after menopause and continues to increase the longer she lives with the lowered estrogen levels of old age.

[26] The findings of the Framingham Study were published in *The New England Journal of Medicine* on February 27, 1997.

[27] Altman, Roberta, *Waking Up, Fighting Back: The Politics of Breast Cancer* (Little, Brown, 1996), p. 88.

[28] "Tobacco, Drug Firms Linked to FDA Critics," Associated Press, *San Francisco Chronicle*, July 24, 1996, p. A4.

[29] Wolf, Naomi, *The Beauty Myth: How Images of Beauty Are Used Against Women* (Morrow, 1991; Anchor Books, 1992).

[30] Cousins, Norman, *Anatomy of an Illness As Perceived by the Patient: Reflections on Healing and Regeneration* (W.W. Norton, 1979), p. 36.

[31] Russell, Sabin, "FDA Moves to Ban an Allergy Drug," San Francisco Chronicle, January 14, 1997, p. A1. Hoechst Marion Roussel agreed to remove Seldane from the market when the FDA approved another drug made by the company, Allegra-D, to replace it. According to Marlene Cimons of the *Los Angeles Times* (December 30, 1997), about 1 million prescriptions for Seldane were written during the time the FDA was trying to get the drug off the market.

[32] An Associated Press story (September 18, 1996) reported that the study done at the University of Virginia failed to find any patients who benefited from the procedure. According to the report, right-heart catheterization was used a million or more times a year in the U.S.

Chapter 9

[33] At Vanderbilt University in the 1940s, some 820 unsuspecting pregnant women were given doses of radioactive iron. In a prison in Oregon and one in Washington from 1963 to 1971, prisoners' testicles were irradiated to see what doses would make them sterile. In a Miami hospital from 1980 to 1982, 500 people were injected with radioactive dye without their permission. Around the time of President Clinton's apology to victims of the Tuskegee Study, there were many newspaper stories detailing other abuses like those mentioned here. On March 29, 1997, the *San Francisco Chronicle* reported that the Clinton administration "announced new measures yesterday that are intended to prevent Americans from ever again becoming unwitting subjects for government medical research."

[34] The story by the *Plain Dealer* was picked up by Reuters news service and published in many newspapers, including the *San Francisco Chronicle* on December 16, 1996.

[35] DeGregorio, Michael W. and Valerie J. Wiebe, *Tamoxifen and Breast Cancer* (Yale University Press, 1995, 1996), p. 95. Since millions of women—some of them cancer patients, some just worried about someday getting breast cancer—are being advised to take the drug tamoxifen, it is important to learn all we can about it. Among the books that discuss the drug and the studies done on it, I found these three most interesting: DeGregorio and Wiebe's *Tamoxifen and Breast Cancer; To Dance with the Devil* by Karen Stabiner (op. cit.), and *Waking Up, Fighting Back* by Roberta Altman (op. cit.).

[36] Cousins, Norman, *The Healing Heart: Antidotes to Panic and Helplessness* (W. W. Norton & Company, 1983), p. 25.

Chapter 10

[37] In her *Breast Book* (p. 380), Dr. Susan Love cites a 10 percent incidence rate. *A Woman's Guide to Breast Cancer Diagnosis and Treatment*, published by the Medical Board of California (p. 15), cuts a wider swath, saying lymphedema strikes "about 5% to 20% of women" after breast surgery or radiation. Both say the condition can occur immediately after treatment or years later.

[38] The general belief that lumpectomy is as effective as mastectomy stems largely from a study conducted by Pittsburgh surgeon Bernard Fisher, which was published in 1985. The study showed a 10 percent local recurrence rate for lumpectomy with radiation and an 8 percent rate for mastectomy. For a good layman's discussion of the study and its results, see *To Dance with the Devil* by Karen Stabiner, op. cit., p. 57.

[39] Stabiner, Karen, *To Dance with the Devil*, op. cit., p. 57.

[40] Love, Susan, with Karen Lindsey, *Dr. Susan Love's Breast Book*, op. cit., p. 402.

[41] Runowicz, Carolyn D., and Donna Haupt, *To Be Alive*, op. cit., pp. 80, 116, 179.

[42] Looking for ways to strengthen the immune system, Simonton did pioneering research on the effectiveness of visualization and biofeedback in cancer patients. He and his wife published their results in 1978, causing tremendous controversy. Their book, now mostly available only in libraries, is fascinating: *Getting Well Again: A Step-by-Step, Self-Help Guide to Overcoming Cancer for Patients and Their Families* by O. Carl Simonton, M.D., Stephanie Matthews-Simonton, and James Creighton (J.P. Tarcher, 1978; Bantam, 1992).

[43] Love, Susan, *Dr. Susan Love's Breast Book,* op. cit., p. 412.

[44] Wadler, Joyce, *My Breast: One Woman's Cancer Story* (Addison Wesley, 1992; Pocket Books, 1994), p. 60 (page citation is to the first edition).

[45] In *To Dance with the Devil*, op. cit. (p. 222), Karen Stabiner estimates that about 120,000 American women each year face this treatment dilemma.

[46] Chopra, Deepak, M.D., *Quantum Healing: Exploring the Frontiers of Mind/Body Medicine* (Bantam, 1989), p. 47.

[47] The Boston Women's Health Book Collective, *The New Our Bodies, Ourselves* (Simon & Schuster, 1984, 1992), pp. 620, 624.

[48] Ibid., p. 620.

[49] Altman, Roberta, *Waking Up, Fighting Back,* op. cit., p. 192.

[50] Stabiner, Karen, *To Dance with the Devil*, op. cit., p. 338.

[51] DeGregorio, Michael W. and Valerie J. Wiebe, *Tamoxifen and Breast Cancer*, op. cit., pp. 55, 57.

[52] Authors Love, Altman, Stabiner, and DeGregorio and Wiebe all discuss the effects and side effects of tamoxifen, as do many other authors of books on breast cancer and its treatment.

[53] Rosenblum, Barbara, and Sandra Butler, *Cancer in Two Voices* (Spinsters Book Company, San Francisco, 1991), p. 23.

Chapter 11

[54] Technically, the word *menopause* refers to the point in time at which a woman permanently stops menstruating. Most women call the whole long, annoying change-of-life process menopause, and that is the sense in which I use the word here.

[55] Barbach, Lonnie, Ph.D. *The Pause: Positive Approaches to Menopause* (Dutton, 1993).

[56] The remedies Ullman has created are unusual in that they address a group of symptoms that appear together, rather than a single symptom. They are sold under the trade name Medicine from Nature. Information on homeopathy is available from Homeopathic Educational Services, 2124 Kittredge St., Berkeley, CA 94704.

[57] Although earlier studies based on consumption of foods rich in beta carotene had positive results, two studies using beta carotene pills turned deadly. In the first, a 10-year study of male smokers in Finland begun in the mid-1980s, subjects who took beta carotene developed 18 percent more lung cancer than those who didn't take the pills. The second study, conducted among smokers in the U.S. by the National Cancer Institute, was shut down in January 1996 when researchers realized there were 28 percent more lung cancers and 17 percent more deaths among those who took the beta carotene (Associated Press, January 19, 1996; May 20, 1997).

[58] Wallis, Claudia, "A Puzzling Plague," *Time*, January 14, 1991, p. 48.

[59] Altman, Roberta, *Waking Up, Fighting Back*, op. cit., p. 53.

[60] Ibid., p. 51.

[61] The study, sometimes referred to as the Harvard-Yale Nurses' study, surveyed nearly 90,000 American nurses about their health and lifestyle. It was completed in 1992. Personally, I am skeptical of its results because information was not gathered from physical examinations, medical records, or even interviews. Instead, subjects were sent mail-in questionnaires.

[62] Brody, Jane E., "Chemicals in Food Called Minimal Cancer Risk," *San Francisco Chronicle*, February 16, 1996, p. A10. The "prestigious scientific panel" was a 20-member panel of the National Research Council, an arm of the National Academy of Sciences. Their report focused on their finding that chemicals in food are not a major cause of disease. The food industry applauded the report, choosing to ignore the finding that some half-million new cancer cases a year in the U.S. are attributable to what and how we eat.

[63] "Study Says Exercise Cuts Risk of Breast Cancer," *San Francisco Chronicle*, May 1, 1997, p. A1. A corroborating study is cited by John Link, M.D., in his book *The Breast Cancer Survival Manual* (Henry Holt, 1998, p. 132). This study, conducted at the University of Southern California and reported in 1994, found that four hours of exercise per week reduces a woman's breast cancer risk by as much as 50 percent.

[64] Stabiner, Karen, *To Dance with the Devil*, op. cit., p. 289.

[65] Results of the study, conducted at University Hospital in Geneva, were published in the *American Journal of Epidemiology* in the spring of 1996, and summarized in the *New York Times* by Jane E. Brody on May 5, 1996. Women in the study who smoked less than half a pack a day doubled their risk of breast cancer. Those who smoked 10 to 19 cigarettes a day increased their risk 2.7 times, and those who smoked a pack or more a day increased their risk 4.6 times. The study also showed a threefold increase in risk among nonsmoking women regularly exposed to tobacco smoke.

[66] Nachtigall, Lila, M.D., and Robert D. Nachtigall, M.D., and Joan Rattner Heilman, *What Every Woman Should Know* op. cit., p. 129.

[67] Perlman, David, "Death Risk From Cigarettes Higher Than Ever, Study Finds," *San Francisco Chronicle*, April 24, 1997, p. A15. Researchers for the National Cancer Institute analyzed five different studies of death rates among more than 2.7 million smokers and nonsmokers. The most frightening statistics showed that between 1959 and 1982 the risk of death from smoking-related lung cancer doubled for men and quadrupled for women. Black women, especially, increase their risk by smoking, according to the study; those who smoke run a 23 times greater risk of fatal lung cancer than those who don't smoke. Among white women, a smoker's risk is 18.6 times greater.

Chapter 12

[68] Runowicz, Carolyn D., M.D., and Donna Haupt, *To Be Alive*, op. cit., p. 19.

[69] Ibid., p. 164.

[70] Chopra, Deepak, M.D., *Quantum Healing*, op. cit., p. 157.

[71] Simonton, O. Carl, M.D., Stephanie Matthews-Simonton, and James Creighton, *Getting Well Again*, op. cit., p. 22.

[72] Moyers, Bill, *Healing and the Mind*, op. cit., p. 159.

[73] Davis, Wade, *The Serpent and the Rainbow* (Simon & Schuster, 1985), p. 161.

[74] Ibid., p. 151.

[75] Hirshberg, Caryle, and Marc Ian Barasch, *Remarkable Recovery*, op. cit., p. 296.

[76] Cousins, Norman, *Anatomy of an Illness as Perceived by the Patient*, op. cit., pp. 46, 59.

[77] Ibid., p. 45.

[78] Sobel, David S., M.D., *Partners in Health*, Spring 1997, p. 5. Sobel is also editor of *Mind/Body Health Newsletter*, in which his article "The Mind/Body Guilt Syndrome" originally appeared (Vol.5, No. 2, 1996).

Chapter 14

[79] Faludi, Susan, *Backlash: The Undeclared War Against American Women* (Crown, 1991), p. xv.

[80] Susan Love's descriptions of reconstruction procedures in her *Breast Book* are as clear, concise, and well illustrated as any I've found. I suggest you read her "Reconstruction" section, which begins on page 387, for a basic understanding of what's involved.

[81] Stabiner, Karen, *To Dance with the Devil*, op. cit., p. 252.

[82] Heller, Joseph, *Catch-22* (Simon & Schuster, 1961).

[83] Faludi, Susan, *Backlash*, op. cit., p. 217.

[84] Ibid., p. 219.

[85] Nachtigall, Lila, M.D., and Robert D. Nachtigall, M.D., and Joan Rattner Heilman, *What Every Woman Should Know*, op. cit., p. 160.

[86] Altman, Roberta, *Waking Up, Fighting Back*, op. cit., p. 249.

[87] Runowicz, Carolyn D., M.D., and Donna Haupt, *To Be Alive*, op. cit., p. 74.

[88] Stabiner, Karen, *To Dance with the Devil*, op. cit., p. 114.

[89] Murphy, Suzanne Zahrt, "There Is No 'Simple' Mastectomy," *San Francisco Chronicle*, February 19, 1997, p. A19.

[90] Altman, Roberta, *Waking Up, Fighting Back*, op. cit., p.5.

[91] Dackman, Linda, *Up Front: Sex and the Post-Mastectomy Woman* (Penguin, 1990), p. 42.

Chapter 15

[92] Ayalah, Daphna, and Isaac J. Weinstock, *Breasts: Women Speak Out About Their Breasts and Their Lives* (Summit Books, 1979), p. 224.

[93] Ibid., p. 224.

Chapter 16

[94] Physicians are sued more often by breast cancer patients than by any other group. A national study conducted by the Physician Insurers Association of America in 1995 concluded that "delayed diagnosis of breast cancer is the most common reason for malpractice claims against physicians" and has

resulted in "the largest indemnity payments of any medical condition in the United States." (Medical Board of California, *Action Report*, October 1998, p. 8.)

[95] Six hundred women aged 20 to 50 participated in the nationwide survey, the results of which were released on October 3, 1997.

[96] "Fear of Cancer Makes Women Ignore Other Killers, Study Says," story by the Associated Press, *San Francisco Chronicle*, November 18, 1997, p. A5. This survey questioned more than 1,000 women aged 45 to 54. Some 61 percent said they fear cancer more than any other sickness, and 24 percent specified breast cancer. Only 9 percent named heart attack as their biggest fear, although heart attacks are the number-one killer of American women.

Chapter 17

[97] Steingraber, Sandra, *Living Downstream: An Ecologist Looks at Cancer and the Environment* (Addison Wesley Longman/Perseus Books, 1997).

[98] Standards for organic foods vary from state to state. California's rules are among the strictest. Find out what an organic label means in your state; in some states there are no enforced standards, so the label doesn't mean anything.

[99] Resistance to chemicals of all kinds is a growing problem in both health care and agriculture. Just as head lice have mutated to resist the poisons we use against them, so have agricultural pests and the bacteria that sicken us. In trying to wipe out our enemies we often end up making them stronger. Sandra Steingraber talks, in *Living Downstream* (op. cit.), of the alarming increase in both the toxicity and the volume of poisons now being used by farmers, while agricultural pests continue to damage crops. Meanwhile, doctors bemoan the fact that overuse of antibiotics has led to a new wave of staph infections that are immune to all known drugs.

[100] In early 1998, increasing consumer demand for organic produce prompted the owners of large U.S. commercial farms to try to change the federal government's definition of "organic" so that they could enter the market, estimated at $4 billion a year. They lobbied the government to allow foods that had been genetically engineered, irradiated, or fertilized with

sewage sludge to be labelled organic. It looked like they would prevail, until protest letters from some 200,000 furious consumers flooded the Agriculture Department. In May 1998, the department declined the request. Federal regulation of organic labeling is new (the first federal standards were proposed in December 1997), and still vulnerable. We must remain vigilant.

Recommended Reading

I read dozens and dozens of books, looking for guidance during my own breast cancer experience and later looking for insights to help me in writing this book. Following is a list of the ones I found most helpful. Often, the books that taught me the most weren't about cancer at all.

Altman, Roberta, *Waking Up, Fighting Back: The Politics of Breast Cancer* (Little, Brown, 1996)
A well-researched book by a medical journalist.

Anderson, Greg, *50 Essential Things To Do When the Doctor Says It's Cancer* (Plume/Penguin, 1993)
Not specifically about breast cancer, but there's some good commonsense advice here. By the founder of The Cancer Conquerers.

Ayalah, Daphna, and Isaac J. Weinstock, *Breasts: Women Speak Out About Their Breasts and Their Lives* (Summit Books, 1979)
A fascinating collection of photos and interviews. Only a few of the women have had cancer, but all shed light on women's wide-ranging attitudes toward our bodies.

Barbach, Lonnie, Ph.D. *The Pause: Positive Approaches to Menopause* (Dutton, 1993)
Many women with breast cancer simultaneously have to cope with menopause, either natural or treatment-induced. This is one of the best menopause books I've found.

The Boston Women's Health Book Collective, *The New Our Bodies, Ourselves* (Simon & Schuster, 1984, 1992)
Offers a positive point of view and good information in sections on cancer in general and breast cancer in particular.

Butler, Sandra, and Barbara Rosenblum, *Cancer in Two Voices* (Spinsters Book Company, 1991)
A personal, poetic account co-authored by a woman dying of breast cancer and her lover. It's powerful, but sad. Read it after you're well again.

Chopra, Deepak, M.D., *Quantum Healing: Exploring the Frontiers of Mind/Body Medicine* (Bantam, 1989)
A fascinating book, although I found some parts too technical and hard to understand.

Cousins, Norman, *Anatomy of an Illness As Perceived by the Patient: Reflections on Healing and Regeneration* (W. W. Norton, 1979)
A brilliant, inspiring book. Cousins was a compelling writer and a very feisty patient.

Cousins, Norman, *The Healing Heart: Antidotes to Panic and Helplessness* (W.W. Norton & Company, 1983)
What the author learned from his heart attack. His wisdom applies just as well to breast cancer.

Dackman, Linda, *Up Front: Sex and the Post-Mastectomy Woman* (Penguin, 1990)
A first-person account of a young woman's struggle to return to social and sexual activity after mastectomy and reconstruction.

Davis, Wade, *The Serpent and the Rainbow* (Simon & Schuster, 1985)
An engrossing account of a Harvard grad student's search for the truth about zombification in Haiti. It provides insight into the connections between belief and the impact of drugs on the body.

It seems to me there are a lot of people these days trying to drive men and women apart. In the past few years a growing number of preachers and therapists, and even a poet or two, have been declaring that men and women should return to their traditional roles, meaning that women should go back to being silent and dominated by men. I doubt that all the chest-beating (and drum-beating) will convince many women to return to the subservient position we held and detested for so long, but I fear it may succeed in setting back the progress men and women have made toward being able to talk to each other.

I'm sure you will be there physically for your partner during her breast cancer crisis, available to drive her to medical appointments and do extra chores so she can rest. That's great, but she needs something more from you, something that requires real strength and maturity. She needs you to be available to her emotionally, ready and willing to listen and to talk about what both of you are really feeling. She needs to know that she can make the decisions that are best for her health without worrying that if her body changes you will turn away from her.

If you're a man whose life has not been touched by breast cancer, it's still important for you to let the woman you love know that her breasts are not the reason you are with her. No one knows why some women get breast cancer and others don't, or who is likely to be stricken, or when. We do know that it's important for every woman to check regularly for signs of trouble. In general, the serious breast cancer cases are those that are found too late, after the cancer has begun to spread to other parts of the body. If your partner believes that losing a breast would mean losing your love, she may refuse to have a mammogram or to do breast self-exams out of fear of finding a lump. By avoiding

A revealing personal memoir by the well-known novelist and editor. Cancer is just as frightening and bewildering to men as it is to women.

Love, Susan M., M.D., with Karen Lindsey, *Dr. Susan Love's Breast Book* (Addison Wesley Longman/Perseus Books, 2nd ed., 1995)
This is probably the best source of medical information on breast cancer for the layman. The explanations of symptoms and treatments are clear and thorough, and it has lots of charts and illustrations.

Moch, Susan Diemert, *Breast Cancer: Twenty Women's Stories* (National League for Nursing Press, 1995)
Personal insights from women who have been there.

Moyers, Bill, *Healing and the Mind* (Doubleday, 1993)
Companion to the PBS television series that explored the interaction of the mental and the physical in health care. Includes an interview with Stanford psychiatrist Dr. David Spiegel.

Murphy, Gerald P., M.D., Lois B. Morris, and Dianne Lange, *Informed Decisions* (Viking, 1997)
The big book of cancer information put out by the American Cancer Society. It should be in your public library.

Myers, Art, *Winged Victory: Altered Images. Transcending Breast Cancer* (photos with poems by Maria Marrocchino) (Photographic Gallery of Fine Art Books, San Diego, 1996)
Women who have had breast cancer and the men in their lives talk about their feelings. Photographs are semi-nude.

Simonton, O. Carl, M.D., Stephanie Matthews-Simonton, and James Creighton, *Getting Well Again: A Step-by-Step, Self-Help Guide to Overcoming Cancer for Patients and Their Families* (J.P. Tarcher; distributed by St.Martin's Press, 1978; Bantam, 1992)
Simonton is a pioneer in the field of mind-body interactions.

Stabiner, Karen, *To Dance with the Devil: The New War on Breast Cancer: Politics, Power, and People* (Delacorte Press, 1997)

A dramatic behind-the-scenes account that focuses on Dr. Susan Love and her breast cancer clinic.

Steinem, Gloria, *Revolution from Within: A Book of Self-Esteem* (Little, Brown, 1992)
Steinem describes her own run-in with breast cancer, which was brief and comparatively uneventful. It did make her stop and reevaluate her life, which is one of the positive things it does for many women.

Steingraber, Sandra, *Living Downstream: An Ecologist Looks at Cancer and the Environment* (Addison Wesley Longman/Perseus Books, 1997)
A frightening study of our poisoned environment and how it is undermining our health. The author was diagnosed with bladder cancer in her twenties.

Stoppard, Dr. Miriam, *The Breast Book: The Essential Guide to Breast Care & Breast Health for Women of All Ages* (DK, 1996)
Some good basic medical explanations, although Stoppard tends to play down the side-effects of standard treatments.

Wadler, Joyce, *My Breast: One Woman's Cancer Story* (Addison Wesley Longman, 1992; Pocket Books, 1994)
A snappy, well-written story by a single New York writer who went through lots of stress in coping with her breast cancer.

Weil, Andrew, M.D. *Spontaneous Healing* (Knopf, 1995)
The bestseller. A fine book, but Weil doesn't say much about cancer.

Wolf, Naomi, *The Beauty Myth* (Doubleday, 1991)
A somewhat strident but important examination of how superficial standards of beauty affect women's lives.

Index

A

activism, 233-243

acupressure, 161

acupuncture, 161

African American women, 22, 253

age and breast cancer, 22-23

alternative therapies, 151-164

Altman, Roberta, 146, 157, 199, 253

American Breast Cancer Awareness
Month, 20

American Cancer Society, 17

anesthesia, 138

anorexia, 8

antibiotics, 102

appearance, 8, 192-206

Asian women, 22

aspirin, 107

assertiveness, 50-52, 103

attitude, positive, 25, 26, 38, 49,
86-96, 166-177

Australia, 171

Ayala, Daphna, 210

B

Bacchus, Patricia Jones, 112

Barasch, Marc Ian, 172

beta carotene, 156, 260

biofeedback, 164, 173, 259

biopsies, 29, 30, 48

bone density, 109

breast cancer, cell growth, 29-31;
diagnosing, 10-12, 22, 37; gene,
108, 253; metastatic, 145, 146;
mortality, 20-22, 252, 254; prognosis, 142-143; psychological and
emotional issues, 1, 11, 12;
research, 233-236; recurrence, 26,
221; risk factors, 21-25, 108-109,
253; statistics, 21-25

MENOPAUSE WITHOUT MEDICINE *New Third Edition*
by Linda Ojeda, Ph.D.

Linda Ojeda broke new ground when she began her study of nonmedical approaches to menopause more than ten years ago. In this update of her classic book, she discusses natural sources of estrogen; how mood swings are affected by diet and personality; and the newest research on osteoporosis, breast cancer, and heart disease. She thoroughly examines the hormone therapy debate; suggests natural remedies for depression, hot flashes, sexual changes, and skin and hair problems. As seen in *Time* magazine.

352 pages ... 40 illus. ... Paperback $14.95 ... Hardcover $23.95

THE NATURAL ESTROGEN DIET: Healthy Recipes for Perimenopause and Menopause
by Dr. Lana Liew with Linda Ojeda, Ph.D.

Two women's health and nutrition experts offer women almost 100 easy and delicious recipes to naturally increase their level of estrogen. Each recipe includes nutritional information such as the calories, cholesterol, and calcium content. They also provide an overview of how estrogen can be derived from the food we eat, describe which foods are the highest in estrogen content, and offer meal plan ideas.

224 pages ... 25 illus. ... Paperback $13.95

HER HEALTHY HEART: A Woman's Guide to Preventing and Reversing Heart Disease Naturally
by Linda Ojeda, Ph.D.

Heart disease is the #1 killer of American women ages 44 to 65, yet most of the research is done on men. *Her Healthy Heart* fills this gap by addressing the unique aspects of heart disease in women and natural ways to combat it. Dr. Ojeda explains how women can prevent heart disease whether they take hormone replacement therapy (HRT) or not. She also provides information on how women can reduce their risk of heart disease by making changes in diet, increasing physical activity, and managing stress. A 50-item lifestyle questionnaire helps women discover areas to work on.

352 pages ... 7 illus. ... Paperback $14.95 ... Hard cover $24.95

To order books see last page or call (800) 266-5592

ORDER FORM

10% DISCOUNT on orders of $50 or more —
20% DISCOUNT on orders of $150 or more —
30% DISCOUNT on orders of $500 or more —
On cost of books for fully prepaid orders

NAME

ADDRESS

CITY/STATE   ZIP/POSTCODE

PHONE   COUNTRY (outside of U.S.)

TITLE	QTY	PRICE	TOTAL
The Feisty Woman's...Book *(paper)*		@ $14.95	
The Feisty Woman's...Book *(hard cover)*		@ $24.95	

Prices subject to change without notice

Please list other titles below:

		@ $	
		@ $	
		@ $	
		@ $	
		@ $	
		@ $	
		@ $	
		@ $	

Shipping Costs:
First book: $3.00 by book post ($4.50 by UPS, Priority Mail, or to ship outside the U.S.)
Each additional book: $1.00
For rush orders and bulk shipments call us at (800) 266-5592

TOTAL
Less discount @_____%   (_____)
TOTAL COST OF BOOKS
Calif. residents add sales tax
Shipping & handling
TOTAL ENCLOSED
Please pay in U.S. funds only

❑ Check ❑ Money Order ❑ Visa ❑ Mastercard ❑ Discover

Card # _____ Exp. date _____

Signature _____

Complete and mail to:
Hunter House Inc., Publishers
PO Box 2914, Alameda CA 94501-0914
Orders: (800) 266-5592   email: ordering@hunterhouse.com
Phone (510) 865-5282 Fax (510) 865-4295
❑ Check here to receive our book catalog

FWB 8/99